Occupational Cancer
in Developing Countries

INTERNATIONAL AGENCY FOR RESEARCH ON CANCER

The International Agency for Research on Cancer (IARC) was established in 1965 by the World Health Assembly, as an independently financed organization within the framework of the World Health Organization. The headquarters of the Agency are at Lyon, France.

The Agency conducts a programme of research concentrating particularly on the epidemiology of cancer and the study of potential carcinogens in the human environment. Its field studies are supplemented by biological and chemical research carried out in the Agency's laboratories in Lyon and, through collaborative research agreements, in national research institutions in many countries. The Agency also conducts a programme for the education and training of personnel for cancer research.

The publications of the Agency are intended to contribute to the dissemination of authoritative information on different aspects of cancer research. A complete list of Agency publications is printed at the back of this book.

Cover illustration: Women employed in the steel plant at Jamshodpur,
State of Bihar, India.
Photo: International Labour Office

WORLD HEALTH ORGANIZATION

INTERNATIONAL AGENCY FOR RESEARCH ON CANCER

INSTITUTE OF OCCUPATIONAL HEALTH, FINLAND

INTERNATIONAL LABOUR OFFICE

Occupational Cancer in Developing Countries

Edited by:

N. Pearce, E. Matos, H. Vainio, P. Boffetta and M. Kogevinas

IARC Scientific Publications No. 129

International Agency for Research on Cancer

Lyon 1994

Published by the International Agency for Research on Cancer,
150 cours Albert Thomas, 69372 Lyon Cedex 08, France

Distributed by Oxford University Press, Walton Street, Oxford OX2 6DP, UK
Distributed in the USA by Oxford University Press, New York

IARC Library Cataloguing in Publication Data

Occupational cancer in developing countries /
  editors, Pearce, N . . . [et al].

  (IARC scientific publications ; 129)

  1. Occupational diseases 2. Neoplasms 3. Developing countries
  I. Pearce, N. II. Series
  ISBN 92 832 2129 X   (NLM Classification: QZ 202)
  ISSN 0300−5085

Printed in the United Kingdom

Contents

Introduction

N. Pearce and E. Matos

Part I.   GENERAL ISSUES

Chapter 1.   Industrialization and health

N. Pearce, E. Matos, M. Koivusalo and S. Wing

Chapter 2.   Transfer of hazardous industries

J. Jeyaratnam

Chapter 8.   Other diseases
E. Matos and P. Boffetta

Part IV.   PRIMARY PREVENTION AND CONTROL

Chapter 9.   International and national measures for prevention and control

Action of WHO
M.I. Mikheev
Action and guidelines of ILO
K. Kurppa and J. Takala
National control measures
E. Matos and C. Partensky

Chapter 10.   Strategies for the prevention of occupational cancer in developing countries
N. Pearce and E. Matos

Appendix: Survey of information on legislation, exposure and industries in developing countries
E. Matos and H. Vainio

Foreword

Cancers due to exposures in the workplace in developing counties have received little attention, in part because of the overriding problems in those regions of communicable diseases, malnutrition and vulnerability to natural disasters. This book shows, however, that the global process of industrialization is resulting in increased exposures to occupational carcinogens in developing countries, owing to unsafe technology or ineffective legislation on occupational safety and health. These factors are exacerbated by the fact that a work-force with poor health and nutritional status, and which includes many women and children, is more vulnerable to many diseases, including cancer. The transfer of hazardous industries and wastes from developed to developing countries is of particular concern.

The importance of this publication is that it brings together in one place all of the available published data on occupational cancer in developing countries. It presents the results of a survey carried out at IARC on common occupational exposures and measures that have been taken to control them. The overview indicates where information is lacking about the health effects of agents used in developing countries, many of which are banned or restricted elsewhere.

It is my hope that this book will stimulate the development of appropriate, effective measures for prevention.

P. Kleihues
Director, IARC

List of authors and affiliations

P. Boffetta, International Agency for Research on Cancer, 150 cours Albert Thomas, 69372 Lyon Cedex 08, France

V. Forastieri, International Labour Organisation, Geneva, Switzerland

J. Jeyaratnam, National University of Singapore, Singapore

M. Kogevinas, International Agency for Research on Cancer, 150 cours Albert Thomas, 69372 Lyon Cedex 08, France (present address: Department of Epidemiology and Public Health, Institut Municipal d'Investigacio Medica, 80 Doctor Aiguader Road, Barcelona 08003, Spain)

M. Koivusalo, Finnish Cancer Registry, Liisankatu 21B, 00170 Helsinki, Finland

K. Kurppa, International Labour Organisation, Geneva, Switzerland

R. Loewenson, Zimbabwe Congress of Trade Unions, Harare, Zimbabwe

E. Matos, International Agency for Research on Cancer, 150 cours Albert Thomas, 69372 Lyon Cedex 08, France (present address: Instituto de Oncologia 'Angel H. Roffo', Av. San Martin 5481, 1417 Buenos Aires, Argentina)

M.I. Mikheev, World Health Organization, 1211 Geneva, Switzerland

C. Partensky, International Agency for Research on Cancer, 150 cours Albert Thomas, 69372 Lyon Cedex 08, France

N. Pearce, International Agency for Research on Cancer, 150 cours Albert Thomas, 69372 Lyon Cedex 08, France (present address: Wellington School of Medicine, Main Street, Newtown, PO Box 7343, Wellington South, Aotearoa, New Zealand

P. Pisani, International Agency for Research on Cancer, 150 cours Albert Thomas, 69372 Lyon Cedex 08, France

J. Takala, International Labour Organisation, Geneva, Switzerland

H. Vainio, International Agency for Research on Cancer, 150 cours Albert Thomas, 69372 Lyon Cedex 08, France (present address: Department of Industrial Hygiene and Toxicology, Institute of Occupational Health, Topeliuksenkatu 41aA, 00250, Helsinki, Finland)

S. Wing, Department of Epidemiology, School of Public Health, University of North Carolina, Chapel Hill, NC 27514, USA

Acknowledgements

This monograph was prepared during 1992−93 at IARC in collaboration with the Finnish Institute of Occupational Health in Helsinki, and with ILO's Technical Cooperation programme, in particular, with the ILO/FINNIDA Asian Regional Programme on Occupational Safety and Health and the ILO/FINNIDA African Safety and Health Project and within the framework of the ILO Programme for the Improvement of Working Conditions and Environment (PIACT).

The project was begun by Elena Matos, who surveyed the situation with regard to occupational cancer in developing countries, drafted many of the chapters and did preliminary editing on others. After Elena Matos returned to Argentina, Neil Pearce completed the editing of the book while at IARC on a Visiting Scientist Award; his work was continued during tenure of a Senior Research Fellowship of the Health Research Council of New Zealand.

Several other members of the IARC staff played important roles in the production of this volume. In particular, Jane Mitchell organized the voluminous correspondence and typed the many drafts of the manuscript. We should also like to thank Rodolfo Saracci, Chief of the Unit of Analytical Epidemiology at IARC, and Lorenzo Tomatis, Director of the Agency, for their support and encouragement.

We also wish to thank the many colleagues who commented on the draft manuscript, including Ricardo Cabral, Meri Koivusalo, Kari Kurppa, Philip J. Landrigan, Jyrki Liesivuori, Enzo Merler, Paola Pisani, Deogratias Sekimpi and Steve Wing. In particular, we received extensive comments from Timo Partanen and Paul Demers. We also wish to thank Prashant Chattopadhyay for his assistance with the literature review and for compiling data on India during his visit to the Agency while holding a UICC ICRETT fellowship, and Marceil Yeater (UNEP) for information on legislation. Finally, we wish to thank Elisabeth Heseltine for editing the manuscript.

Neil Pearce, Elena Matos, Harri Vainio,
Paolo Boffetta, Manolis Kogevinas
Lyon, France
August 1993

Introduction

N. Pearce and E. Matos

Background

The populations of many developing countries are at risk of dying from undernutrition, periodic famines, floods, wars and communicable diseases. It is thus not surprising that relatively little attention has been paid to the problem of occupational cancer, often regarded as being primarily a problem of industrialized countries. Since, however, imported manufacturing processes often meet with an institutional infrastructure different from that for which they were designed and a work-force that may be particularly vulnerable to exposure to toxic and carcinogenic hazards because of general poor health and malnutrition, there is an increasing need for information about occupational cancer in developing countries. The situation is exacerbated by ineffective legislation for occupational safety and health, nonenforcement of regulations, poor labelling, inadequate supervision, dangerous work practices, unsafe technology and lack of use of protective clothing, in the context of rapid global industrialization and rapid demographic changes.

The developing countries of the Third World are usually considered to be those of Africa, Central and South America, Asia (excluding Japan and the former USSR) and Oceania (excluding Australia and New Zealand) (Parkin, 1986). These areas account for more than 70% of the world's population (see Figure 1), more than 70% of the global land mass and about 70% of the world's work-force. Although the term 'developing countries' is used throughout this book, the terminology is questionable because of the tendency to equate 'development' with 'industrialization' (see Chapter 1) and because it covers a heterogeneous group of countries with divergent social, cultural and political organizations. The situation has become considerably more complex in recent years, as some Asian countries are now highly industrialized and some eastern European countries are relatively less industrialized.

While anecdotal information is available concerning many countries, very few studies have been conducted of exposure to occupational carcinogens in developing countries, and even fewer studies have examined the health consequences of such exposures. There is, however, growing concern that the health impact of many chemicals used in the developing world has been underestimated. This monograph is intended to bring together the information that is currently available.

1

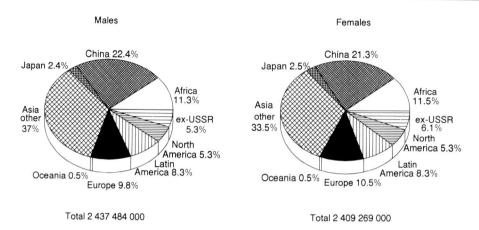

Figure 1. World population estimates, 1980

Format of the monograph

The monograph is divided into four sections: general issues, exposure, health effects and primary prevention and control.

The monograph begins with two chapters which review general issues of industrialization and health. It is argued (Chapter 1) that industrialization has brought mixed benefits, in that it has been accompanied by improved health in some populations but slow improvement or actual deterioration of health in other populations, such as those that provided the labour and raw materials needed for industrialization. Thus, although industrialization may be accompanied by gains in life expectancy, it also has major health costs, including an increased risk for occupational cancer. A particularly relevant issue is the transfer of hazardous industries from developed to developing countries (Chapter 2). These general considerations are followed by an overview of the incidence of occupationally related cancers in developing countries (Chapter 3) and a review of current knowledge about carcinogenic occupational exposures (Chapter 4).

Available information on exposure to occupational carcinogens is reviewed in Part II. In those industries in developing countries for which measurements have been made, the levels of exposure generally exceed the regulatory levels established for industrialized countries (Chapter 5). Exposures may be especially high in some small-scale industries, in which working conditions, hygiene and safety measures are often poor; furthermore, child labour is still commonplace, and children are not covered by safety legislation that applies only to people who are legally employed (Chapter 6).

Part III contains reviews of studies of occupational cancer in developing countries (Chapter 7) and of studies of other diseases caused by occupational carcinogens (Chapter 8), as the occurrence of such diseases implies high levels of exposure. Very little information is available on the occurrence of occupational cancer in developing countries; however, limited information is available on several recognized carcinogens, including asbestos, silica, benzene and ionizing radiation, and various industries, including mining, metal work, the rubber industry, the textile industry and agriculture. Furthermore, asbestosis and silicosis have been found repeatedly in studies of occupationally exposed populations in developing countries.

Part IV contains reviews of preventive action at the international and national levels (Chapter 9) and general strategies for the prevention of occupational cancer in developing countries (Chapter 10). Despite the considerable obstacles to occupational cancer prevention, the situation in most industrialized countries generally continues to improve. The improvement in occupational hygiene standards in industrialized countries has, however, partly (or largely) been achieved by the transfer of hazardous industries to developing countries. Just as the reasons for this transfer are political and economic, substantial progress in the prevention of occupational cancer in developing countries is most likely to come from political and economic change. Nevertheless, there is much that can be achieved, even in the current international situation.

Sources of information

The monograph is primarily a review of previously published information. In addition, a survey was carried out to obtain more information on regulations, policies and common occupational exposures in developing countries (see Appendix). The findings of the survey and of the literature review were useful not only in summarizing current knowledge but also in indicating what is not known. Very little information is available about the levels of exposure or the health effects of the many occupational carcinogens currently in use in developing countries, some of which have been banned or restricted in developed countries.

Concluding remarks

Although this report attempts to give an overview of the situation in developing countries, it should be stressed that it is difficult, and inappropriate, to draw general conclusions about regions with divergent social, economic and political conditions. It is to be hoped that this book will serve not only as a useful summary of currently available knowledge but also to identify major areas in which information is lacking and to motivate the systematic collection of further information on exposure levels and health effects. In addition, we hope that this book will create greater awareness of the problems of occupational cancer in developing countries and further the development of appropriate, effective strategies for prevention.

Reference

Parkin, D.M., ed. (1986) *Cancer Occurrence in Developing Countries* (IARC Scientific Publications No. 75), Lyon, IARC

Part I

General Issues

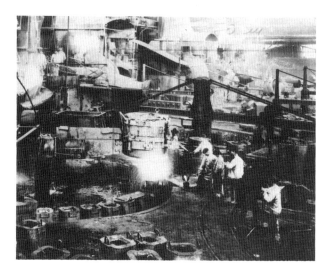

Above: The industrial revolution led to heavy exposure of large populations of workers to substances of quite unknown hazard.

Below: Industrialization in developing countries often involves high exposures to known hazardous substances, because of lack of protective measures and awareness of risk.

Photos: Courtesy of International Labour Office

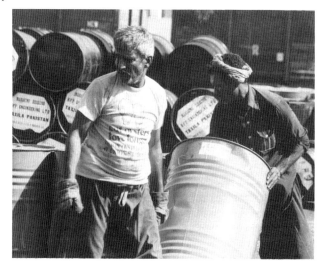

Chapter 1. Industrialization and Health

N. Pearce, E. Matos, M. Koivusalo and S. Wing

Industrialization has been associated with contradictory trends in international health. On the one hand, the countries of Europe and North America which underwent industrialization in the eighteenth and nineteenth centuries have experienced major improvements in average life expectancy, as reflected in the striking relationship between per-capita income, gross national product and life expectancy (Tomatis, 1992). On the other hand, while increased wealth and improved living conditions have been accompanied by improved health in some parts of the population, conditions among the people who have provided the labour and raw materials needed for industrialization have improved more slowly or actually deteriorated. Thus, there are still major, and in some cases increasing, inequalities in income and health in industrialized countries, which can have a significant impact on national mortality rates (Wilkinson, 1992). Very large differentials in health and social conditions are also seen between the industrialized countries and the former colonial world, which is still a source of cheap labour and raw materials (Loewenson, 1993). While little information is available on the effects of socioeconomic differences on health status in developing countries, apart from extensive evidence with regard to absolute poverty, malnutrition and health, such differences appear, if anything, to be greater within the developing countries than within the industrialized countries (Tomatis, 1992).

The industrial revolution

The industrial revolution in Europe initially involved widespread social and economic disruption, unemployment, homelessness, pollution and increased exposure to health hazards both at work and at home. The conditions of factory workers in England during the height of the industrial revolution in the mid-nineteenth century were vividly described by a number of contemporary observers, including Sir Edwin Chadwick, Thomas Carlyle and Friedrich Engels. For example, a physician's report on conditions in Manchester in the 1840s (Engels, 1845) noted that:

> Most travellers are struck by the lowness of stature, the leanness and the paleness which present themselves so commonly to the eye at Manchester, and above all, among the factory classes. ... The men wear out very early in consequence of the conditions under which they live and work. Most of them are unfit for work at forty years, a few hold out to forty-five, almost none to fifty years of age.

As a result of such conditions, the death rate in the United Kingdom and other countries in the first half of the nineteenth century actually increased, before it eventually began to decline in the twentieth century (McKeown, 1988). McKeown (1988) documented the dramatic decline in mortality during the past century from the 'diseases of poverty' that were dominant in the nineteenth century—particularly infectious diseases, respiratory diseases and accidents. The decline in mortality from infectious diseases occurred largely prior to the introduction of effective modern vaccines and treatments and has been attributed mainly to improvements in housing, nutrition and sanitation (Doll, 1992). Such improvements were indirect consequences of general improvements in the standard of living and were due partly to direct governmental and industrial policy: disease and destitution, by injuring and killing workers, interfered with industrial production and put profit in jeopardy; furthermore, infectious diseases were spreading from poor to rich districts (Tomatis, 1992).

The age of development

For the world outside Europe, North America and Oceania, the 'age of development' has been the last 40 years. The 'development' doctrine was proclaimed in the inaugural speech of US President Harry Truman in 1949, who defined most of the world as 'underdeveloped areas' (Sachs, 1990). Development was seen as a linear process, in which certain countries were more 'advanced' than others, and the degree of 'civilization' of a country was measured by the level of its production. Furthermore, developing countries were seen as undergoing the same process experienced by western countries during the industrial revolution, only at a delayed pace. Continued development would be achieved through transfer of technology, western values and investment from the industrialized to the developing countries.

The concept of 'development' has subsequently been the subject of considerable controversy and has been through a number of metamorphoses, including 'social and economic development', 'another development', 'human-centred development', 'integrated development', 'endogenous development', 'redevelopment' and 'sustainable development' (Esteva, 1992). Despite continued attempts to emphasize a distinction between 'industrialization' and 'development', which has as its goal the overall well-being of the people, development policies have frequently equated 'development' with 'economic growth', and particularly with industrialization.

It has been argued (e.g. Sachs, 1990) that the vision of 'development' as synonymous with industrialization paralleled moves to replace the political domination of colonial times with the economic domination of 'anti-colonial imperialism', which encouraged the joint processes of political independence and economic dependence. Even when narrowly conceived in terms of 'industrialization', development has not been a linear process but rather a complex global process in which the industrialization of western countries was based partly on the dependence of countries in the periphery. For example, Mazuri (1986) argued that: 'In the last three centuries, Africa has helped substantially in the building of the West's industrial civilization, while the West may have hampered the evolution of Africa's own industrial culture. Africa's contribution to the West's industrialization has ranged from the era of the slave trade for Western plantations to the new era of cobalt and chrome for Western factories.' In this sense, industrialized and developing countries can be regarded as complementary participants in an overall global process of industrialization.

Thus, the term 'developing countries' is of questionable validity and reflects western concepts of development. Furthermore, as noted above, 'developing countries' do not constitute a uniform block. Although in many countries industrialization has been associated with an increase in per-capita income and improvements in nutrition (Noweir, 1986), major inequalities in wealth remain and in some instances have increased. In some countries an increase in gross national product has been accompanied by little benefit in terms of health, whereas some relatively poor countries (e.g. China, Jamaica, Costa Rica) have made major improvements in health care and life expectancy (Sen, 1988). Clearly, the way in which the gross national product is 'shared' is as important as its absolute level (Wilkinson, 1992); furthermore, health can itself affect economic growth (Behrman, 1993).

Given the experience of the industrial revolution of the nineteenth century, it is not surprising that industrialization has also had some major detrimental effects on health in developing countries. Attitudes to industrialization in the developing countries have changed in recent decades. In many of those countries, industrialization had been viewed as the key means for modernizing society and reducing dependence (Jeyaratnam, 1985). Thus, in the 1970s, the general view was that industrial pollution —which was a major concern of developed countries—was not a major concern for developing countries, that poverty was the main polluter and that industrialization was essential to overcome poverty and improve the standard of living. By the 1980s, the attitudes of industrialized and developing countries had moved closer together, largely as a result of experiences of problems of pollution, occupational disease, social instability and large-scale industrial accidents in developing countries (Tolba & El-Kholy, 1992).

The debt crisis and structural adjustment programmes

Nevertheless, significant progress was made in education and health in many developing countries during the 1960s and 1970s. For example, with political independence, many African governments implemented policies to enable more equitable access to education and health care, some degree of land reform, improved access to water and sanitation, and improved labour policies (Kanji *et al.*, 1991). Even in those countries where the changes were modest, and despite continuing inequalities, significant improvements were made in terms of indicators such as average life expectancy and infant mortality rates. The percentage of the African population who had received primary education doubled between 1960 and 1980, from 36 to 79%; progress was made in health care, control of infectious diseases and access to hospitals, rural clinics and community trained health workers, and child mortality more than halved during 1960–90 (Logie & Woodroffe, 1993).

These benefits faded, however, with the advent of the Third World debt crisis in the 1980s (Alubo, 1990). The debt crisis grew out of the oil crisis of the 1970s, which created large pools of 'petrodollars'; commercial banks then encouraged governments and entrepreneurs in larger developing economies to take large loans (underwritten by the State), while the World Bank and the International Monetary Fund lent money to poorer countries (Smith & Stott, 1992). Much of these funds went to the purchase of arms, returned to foreign bank accounts or went to programmes that had little relation to social or economic development. For example, it has been estimated that in Latin America 92% of the debt was used for capital flight, debt service and the building of dollar reserves, and only 8% was invested domestically (Chernomas, 1990). Nevertheless, real interest rates were low, and export earnings appeared to be high enough to repay the loans of most developing countries. The real crisis came in the 1980s, when monetarist policies were adopted on a global scale, international interest rates soared and commodity prices plunged, leaving most developing countries unable to pay their debts (Kanji *et al.*, 1991). The situation was exacerbated by the continuing flight of capital from developing countries, which accounted, for example, for 70% of all new loans in Latin America since 1982 (Chernomas, 1990).

Although the debtor countries paid more than US$ 1300 billion during 1982–90, they now owe 61% more money than they did in 1982 (Logie & Woodroffe, 1993). In spite of increasing poverty, African countries transfer US$ 10 billion a year to the industrialized countries in debt repayment. The minor benefits that have been obtained in terms of cancellation and rescheduling of debts have been gained at the cost of accepting 'structural adjustment' programmes mandated by the World Bank and the International Monetary Fund. These programmes have included privatization of publicly owned industries, removal of trade and investment controls, currency devaluation, reductions in public borrowing, expenditure and services, removal of food subsidies, deregulation of labour laws, wage freezes, retrenchment, and introduction of school and medical fees.

Although some countries outside of Africa and Latin America that were undergoing structural adjustment programmes experienced growth and improved social conditions during the 1980s, most countries (particularly those in sub-Saharan Africa and Latin America) experienced falling incomes, increasing unemployment, reduced investment and increasing inflation (Onimode, 1989; Stewart, 1991). Thus, some critics have argued that structural adjustment programmes are designed primarily to benefit industrialized countries, by freeing up markets, increasing their access to cheap raw materials, and ensuring that the debt is repaid (Logie & Woodroffe, 1993). With regard to Africa, Kanji *et al.* (1991) argue that the programmes are already reversing the gains that resulted from the overthrow of colonial domination. They quote a former senior manager of the World Bank, as follows:

> I think that under the adjustment label what the Bank and the Fund have really been doing in Africa is to attempt fundamental change in the development paradigm; essentially to convince African governments through the guise of adjustment that their particular form of collectivism, of a type of socialist mixed economy is unworkable.

Under the structural adjustment programmes, government expenditures on health services have decreased (Pinstrup-Andersen, 1993), and the effects have been far-reaching in terms of health, education and nutrition. For example, during the 1960s, nearly all children in the United Republic of Tanzania attended primary school, and life expectancy had reached 60 years; in 1986, after the International Monetary Fund insisted on devaluation of the currency, 60% of all exports were devoted to debt servicing, free schooling had stopped, and the price of maize and rice had increased markedly (Logie, 1992). In Ghana, health care fees rose by 800–1000% in 1985 (Aniyam, 1989).

Infant mortality is particularly sensitive to socioeconomic change; although the rate of infant mortality has improved in most countries over the last few decades (Roemer & Roemer, 1990), in many countries undergoing structural adjustment programmes the rate of improvement has declined or even reversed. Africa is now the only continent in which infant and child mortality is increasing (Summerfield, 1989), and UNICEF reported in 1991 that at least half a million children worldwide had died as a direct result of debt (Logie, 1992).

Structural adjustment programmes have exerted particular pressure on women, in each of their four roles — as producers, home managers, mothers and community organizers (Stewart, 1991). More time is taken in order to earn income outside the home, whereas decreasing household resources necessitate more time for household management (for example, in Lusaka, women produce 50% of the food in low-income households), and deteriorating health and health facilities mean that more time must be spent caring for sick family members.

The scale of the social problems resulting from structural adjustment programmes has led to changes in emphasis in recent years. In particular, UNICEF has called for 'adjustment with a human face' (Cornia *et al.*, 1987), and the Managing Director of the International Monetary Fund (quoted by Stewart, 1991) acknowledged that:

> ... macroeconomic policies can have strong effects on the distribution of income and on social equity and welfare. A responsible adjustment programme must take these effects into account, particularly as they impinge on the most vulnerable or disadvantaged groups in society.

In a detailed review of the changing views of the International Monetary Fund and the World Bank, Stewart (1991) concluded, however, that there had been much change in rhetoric but little action. The few attempts at 'poverty alleviation' had been largely independent of, and peripheral to, structural adjustment programmes and had reached only a limited number of people, who did not belong to the poorest sections of society.

Introduction of new technology and materials

Thus, although the problems of industrialization in developing countries are to some extent analogous to those experienced in European countries, there are some important differences. Furthermore, the industrial revolution in Europe was a gradual process in which mechanization slowly spread as a result of new inventions and discoveries. As the resulting changes in production processes took a long time to develop and to introduce, some opportunity was provided for adaptation (Noweir, 1986). In developing countries, although the pattern of industrialization has varied greatly and is still changing, it has generally been a rapid process. Industrialized countries have nearly 200 years of experience with industrial processes and chemicals, whereas developing countries often have only a few decades (Christiani *et al.*, 1990).

The rapidity of industrialization has permitted little time for adjustment and for training a work-force for the new technologies and production processes. High technology industries (such as the chemical industry) pose significant hazards to a relatively young, untrained work-force (Christiani *et al.*, 1990). In many developing countries, rapid changes have occurred unevenly, and the juxtapositions of old and new, impoverished and high technology are striking; it has been argued therefore that the rapid introduction of the work methods necessary for high technology alongside traditional methods has resulted in considerably higher rates of industrial injuries and occupational diseases in developing countries than in similar industries and processes in industrialized countries (Noweir, 1986).

The problems are exacerbated by the selective transfer of hazardous industries and chemicals to developing countries (see Chapter 2), often in the absence of any information on the risks involved in their use (Castleman, 1979; Simonato, 1986; Huncharek, 1993). For example, more than 50 million pounds (2268 tonnes) of pesticides that are either banned, restricted or unregistered in the USA (such as chlordane, Mirex, Dicofol and dibromochloropropane) were shipped in 1990 from the USA to developing countries, and in particular to those of Latin America (Smith & Beckmann, 1991; Tomatis, 1992). Toxic epidemics have become a serious problem during the twentieth century (Ferrer & Cabral, 1991): the Economic and Social Commission of Asia and the Pacific estimated that up to two million incidents of poisoning by pesticides occur each year throughout the world, of which 40 000 may be fatal (Forget, 1991).

The tendency for hazardous industries to be transferred to developing countries was strengthened by the debt crisis and structural adjustment programmes. A memorandum from the chief economist of the World Bank, dated 12 December 1991 (quoted in *The Economist* [Anon., 1992]), argued that:

> Just between you and me, shouldn't the World Bank be encouraging more migration of the dirty industries to the LDCs [less developed countries]? I can think of three reasons:
>
> 1) The measurement of the costs of health-impairing pollution depends on the forgone earnings from increased morbidity and mortality. From this point of view a given amount of health-impairing pollution should be done in the country with the lowest cost, which will be the country with the lowest wages. I think the economic logic behind dumping a load of toxic waste in the lowest-wage country is impeccable and we should face up to that.
>
> 2) The costs of pollution are likely to be non-linear as the initial increments of pollution probably have very low cost. I've always thought that under-populated countries in Africa are vastly *under*-polluted; their air quality is probably vastly inefficiently low [*sic*] compared to Los Angeles or Mexico City. Only the lamentable facts that so much pollution is generated by non-tradable industries (transport, electrical generation) and that the unit transport costs of solid waste are so high prevent world-welfare-enhancing trade in air pollution and waste.
>
> 3) The demand for a clean environment for aesthetic and health reasons is likely to have very high income-elasticity. The concern over an agent that causes a one-in-a-million change in the odds of prostate cancer is obviously going to be much higher in a country where people survive to get prostate

cancer than in a country where under-5 mortality is 200 per thousand. Also, much of the concern over industrial atmospheric discharge is about visibility-impairing particulates. These discharges may have very little direct health impact. Clearly trade in goods that embody aesthetic pollution concerns could be welfare-enhancing. While production is mobile, the consumption of pretty air is a non-tradable.

The problem with the arguments against all of these proposals for more pollution in LDCs (intrinsic rights to certain goods, moral reasons, social concerns, lack of adequate markets, etc) could be turned around and used more or less effectively against every Bank proposal for liberalization.

Although the memorandum was subsequently described as 'sardonic' and was never taken seriously, it does provide an extreme example of the logic of structural adjustment measures which increase environmental pollution and worsen working conditions.

Local infrastructure

A related problem is incompatibility of imported industries with local infrastructure. Technological development has been accompanied by massive social changes, and developing and newly industrialized countries are now facing the diseases that characterize industrialized societies (such as cardiovascular disease, respiratory disease and cancer) at a time when many of them are still dealing with malnutrition and diseases such as cholera, tuberculosis, malaria and diarrhoea. Thus, established national infrastructures may not respond adequately to the health effects of imported technologies that affect the most vulnerable sections of the population (who are already affected by poverty and malnutrition); few managerial resources are available to assess and manage the hazards, databases are inadequate, and expertise to analyse the consequences of industrial processes to human beings and ecosystems is in short supply (Kasperson & Kasperson, 1987).

In particular, rapid industrialization has not been accompanied by parallel progress in establishing occupational health services (Christiani, 1988). These are usually absent or inadequate, particularly in rural areas, where pesticides may be sprayed in considerable amounts. The lack of such services is due partly to the inevitable delay in educating and training professionals, since resources for training are scarce and professional personnel are attracted by the higher salaries in developed countries. These problems also occur, however, because the rapid development of new forms of ownership and management has outstripped the development of procedures to regulate the new working conditions.

Such problems do not merely involve lack of education and training. The currently increasing sales of tobacco in developing countries demonstrate that hazardous substances may be introduced and promoted even when their health effects are well known (Barry, 1991). In the occupational context, in particular, health and safety do not appear to have been priorities for integration into economic development on a level with productivity and profitability (Quinn *et al.*, 1987). Thus, even when protective technology becomes available, it may be regarded as a production tool rather than as a means to protect workers (McConnell *et al.*, 1992). Specific problems faced by the occupational health services in developing countries include (Noweir, 1986): shortages of professional personnel, facilities and resources; the fact that most enterprises involve agriculture, small industries and seasonal work; administrative and technical limitations; lack of communication and public information; and inadequate legislation. Other, related problems include the inadequacy or absence of safety committees, inadequate labour inspection and weak unions. The latter issue is particularly important, since the strength of worker organizations appears to be one of the main factors that influence the provision of adequate occupational health and safety measures (Elling, 1986).

All of these problems are compounded by the fact that most production workers in developing countries are engaged in the informal sector of the economy, which operates largely outside the system of government benefits and regulations (Christiani et al., 1990). Whereas occupational health services and a regulatory structure may exist in the formal sector, they are rarely present in the informal sector (Lukindo, 1993), which involves a mixture of old and new types of production, diverse processes in small units and weak labour organization. Another factor is that a relatively high proportion of workers come from the most vulnerable sections of the population, including the very young, the very old and women of child-bearing age. (The situation with regard to child labour is reviewed in Chapter 6.)

Social and environmental effects of industrialization

Industrialization affects the environment in three general ways (Tolba & El-Kholy, 1992): by the release of pollutants, by the creation of products that replace environmentally sound traditional products and by the destruction and transformation of natural resources to obtain raw materials. Industrialization not only directly affects workers employed in new industries but also has a considerable impact on the environment, economy, culture and health of the regions in which it is established (Packard, 1989; WHO, 1992) by disrupting the ecological balance, spreading infectious disease and undermining and impoverishing traditional society (Christiani et al., 1990). Industrialization has therefore particularly affected the environment and health of indigenous people, including those in many 'western' countries (Pomare & de Boer, 1988; Bullard, 1993).

In agriculture, the economic pressures that lead to the development of cash crops mean that traditional industry and subsistence agriculture are undermined, resulting in rural impoverishment, landlessness and extensive migratory labour (Loewenson, 1988; Christiani et al., 1990). For example, large portions of land in Latin America that were used for production for local consumption have been reallocated for export-orientated agriculture; as a result, over 40% of the Central American work-force has been estimated to be seasonal migrants (Michaels et al., 1985).

A number of studies have suggested that agricultural irrigation can result in higher densities of parasites and vectors. If adequate sanitation measures are not provided, high rates of schistosomiasis may occur among irrigation workers (Lanoix, 1958), which may account for 12–15% of all cases of bladder cancer in endemic areas (Taba, 1981). Similarly, the expansion of rice-growing areas in Kenya and of cocoa-growing areas in Ghana has contributed to the spread of malaria (Desowitz, 1976). Parasitic diseases are known to aggravate the toxicity of a wide variety of chemicals, even at low levels (WHO, 1981; El Batawi, 1986). For example, a review of autopsies performed on South African miners between 1953 and 1970 revealed that 32% of blacks with evidence of chronic pulmonary fibrotic disease related to heavy exposure to silica (silicosis) also had evidence of active tuberculosis (WHO, 1983). Industries such as mining can further contribute to the spread of communicable diseases: by attracting a concentrated work-force from a variety of regions, by providing living conditions that increase susceptibility to disease and by then repatriating those who become ill (Zengeya *et al.*, 1982). In the same way, industries that use migrant labour also contribute to the spread of communicable diseases (Kloos *et al.*, 1981; Laurel, 1981; Packard, 1989).

Another example of the indirect costs of agricultural development on health is provided by the history of agricultural irrigation in the Awash Valley of Ethiopia (Packard, 1989). The Valley was occupied by a number of semi-nomadic, pastoral ethnic groups, who were evicted to make way for the large-scale cultivation of cotton and sugar (Kloos, 1982). Subsequent construction of dams forced the pastoralists onto less fertile regions of the Valley, which became overgrazed. The nutrition and health of this population declined, and they became more susceptible to the effects of major droughts. They eventually moved to become permanent farm labourers near the irrigation schemes, where there was a high prevalence of parasitic infections (Packard, 1989).

Even when such large-scale developments do not displace smallholders, they may reduce their ability to earn an income from farming (Mandal & Gosh, 1976; Loewenson, 1988). Wisner (1980) suggested that the marginalization of smallholders in eastern Kenya led to a deterioration in childhood nutrition. A similar pattern was observed in Colombia (Taussig, 1978), and large-scale production was identified as a risk factor for infant mortality in Brazil (Victoria & Blank, 1980). Marginalization also produces a drift to urban areas, as the dispossessed search for employment, and the resulting growth of the pool of urban poor creates high risks in terms of infection, disease and violent deaths (Testa Tambellini, 1993). Furthermore, as in western countries in the nineteenth century, massive migration to urban centres and the consequent unemployment or underemployment of large sectors of the population results in competition for jobs among a large, unskilled work-force and therefore a worsening of general working conditions, particularly with regard to health and safety. Urban employment involves additional health hazards, including road accidents during commuting (Cordova *et al.*, 1986).

Installation of new industries also implies a number of direct costs to environmental health in the communities in which they are based. The experience of Bhopal, India, in which a massive leak of methyl isocyanate gas left thousands dead or permanently disabled, probably provides the best illustration of the potential health costs of industrialization (Castleman & Purkavastha, 1985). A number of other examples can be cited, in terms of both routine environmental pollution and catastrophic accidents. Effects of exposure to asbestos have been observed in populations of districts in southern Africa in which asbestos mines are located (Packard, 1989). An epidemic of mercury poisoning occurred in Nicaragua (Hassan *et al.*, 1981) when a chloralkali plant operated over a period of 12 years by an American-based multinational company, Electro-Quimica Pennwalt, Inc., discharged an estimated 40 tonnes of mercury into a lake that serves as the source of drinking-water for Managua and a major source of fish (Ives, 1985). Similarly, a study of children in Kingston, Jamaica (Matte *et al.*, 1989), showed that blood lead levels were significantly higher among children living near repair shops in which scrap lead was smelted. A study in the town of Obuasi in Ghana (Amasa, 1975) showed that both workers in the local gold-mine and townspeople who did not work at the mine had high levels of arsenic in their hair; the vegetation 4 km from the mine, some food items and soil were also found to have unusually high arsenic contents. In Zimbabwe, signs of exposure to organophosphate pesticides were found in workers other than sprayers on large farms, and a high proportion of poisoning cases were in women and children (Bwititi *et al.*, 1987; Loewenson, 1991). Mexican researchers described chromate pollution from a Bayer affiliate near Mexico City, where wastes were piled beside the factory and were used to fill potholes in the streets; children in the neighbourhood developed painful sores (Castleman, 1985). In a review of data from 63 countries for the period 1967−80, Wimberley (1990) concluded that multinational penetration had had significant, harmful effects on infant mortality, although this had been offset to some extent by increased health spending.

Population vulnerability to occupational cancer

The social and environmental effects of industrialization on health are not only a major concern in themselves but are also relevant to occupational cancer, since the hazards of exposure to occupational carcinogens in developing countries depend not only on the level of exposure but also on the vulnerability of the exposed populations (Ong *et al.*, 1993). Subclinical deficiencies in the intake of vitamins A and C were observed in South African miners whose serum vitamin A levels decreased significantly during the first four to six months of service, while there was no clinical evidence of deficiency (Visagie *et al.*, 1974). In a national survey of oesophageal cancer in South African gold-miners, 80% of patients had evidence of past childhood protein−energy malnutrition, and a further 78% had musculoskeletal deformities due to rickets. The areas in which cases were most prevalent were demarcated by the widespread occurrence of nutritional deficiencies (Bradshaw *et al.*, 1982).

Such findings are of concern, since nutritional factors can be an important determinant of subsequent toxicity and carcinogenicity. In particular, low intake of vitamin A and β-carotene, or low intake of foods rich in these vitamins, has been associated with increased risks for cancers at different sites, including lung, larynx, mouth, oesophagus, stomach and urinary bladder (Tomatis *et al.*, 1990). An inverse relationship has been demonstrated between the intake of fresh fruits and vegetables and cancers at various sites, particularly epithelial cancers (Steinmetz & Potter, 1991). It is also known that vitamin deficiencies, common in poor parts of developing countries, can alter the biotransformation of toxicants, and thus their toxicity (WHO, 1981).

Industrialization, politics and health

The contradictory aspects of industrialization discussed above are not unique to developing countries (Brown, 1976). As mentioned above, socioeconomic differences in health have, if anything, increased in industrialized countries in the past century (Marmot & McDowell, 1986; Pearce *et al.*, 1991; Pappas *et al.*, 1993), and there are also large regional differences: black men in Harlem (New York City) are less likely to reach the age of 65 than men in Bangladesh (McCord & Freeman, 1990), and some 'diseases of poverty' such as cholera, tuberculosis and diarrhoea are beginning to return (Spence *et al.*, 1993). Industrialized countries continue to have problems of environmental contamination (Landrigan, 1992). Global environmental changes (including the 'greenhouse effect') associated with industrialization and increasing consumption have transnational results and have 'the ominous capacity to erode the biosphere's carrying capacity for the human—and many other—species' (McMichael, 1993).

The health costs of the process of industrialization are particularly acute in developing countries. Such costs are often viewed as unintentional (and unforeseen) costs of development (e.g. Hunter & Hughes, 1970) which could be largely eliminated, given appropriate knowledge. An alternative approach is to regard health problems as an inevitable cost of production; regulation of toxic and hazardous substances is thus presented as a luxury that poor countries cannot afford. For example, economists from Cubatão (Brazil), one of the most polluted valleys in the world, declared that 'Industry is a necessary evil. ... It is the economic price the undeveloped countries must pay.' (quoted by Navarro, 1984).

Packard (1989) stated that:

> The absence of adequate safety equipment or sanitation standards, the lack of procedures for monitoring former employees for the effects of long term exposure to toxic substances, the absence of worker education about risks of these substances, the squeezing out of small scale producers to meet the needs of internationally based agri-businesses, are frequently the result of hard economic calculations in which production and profit levels are given paramount importance, even though the results of these calculations are often justified in terms of the 'development needs' of the host country.

He therefore argues that the health costs of industrialization cannot be reduced simply by providing knowledge and resources, since appropriate measures to protect health and safety involve costs that neither business nor the state will bear unless it can be seen as being in their interest to do so. Changes are needed in the economic relationships between developing and industrialized countries (Summerfield, 1989), and strong worker organizations should be set up in developing countries (Michaels *et al.*, 1985; Elling, 1988).

The concept of development must be re-examined continually; development must be measured in terms of health and human beings as well as in economic terms and should encompass the overall well-being of the people rather than just that of the financial markets. The World Bank (1989) admitted that: 'Measuring development in terms of access to basic health services, education and food is more satisfactory than using most other yardsticks. Social indicators such as life expectancy reflect more accurately the condition of most of the population than per capita income.'

Concluding remarks

Industrialization has thus been associated with contradictory international trends in health, with some populations (mostly in industrialized countries) experiencing improved services and health and others (mostly in developing countries) seeing slower improvements or even deteriorating conditions as a result of the global process of industrialization. The situation in the countries where the latter populations are found is characterized by (i) the magnitude of the informal sector; (ii) large numbers of workers, including contract workers, who have little or no support from unions or other worker organizations; (iii) the transfer to them of hazardous industries from industrialized countries; (iv) the substitution of export crops for local food crops; (v) insecure status of workers, owing to large-scale unemployment, migratory labour and child labour; (vi) a lack of legislative protection, or the poor enforcement of such protection; and (vii) increasing multinational penetration and decreasing national control over resources.

Overlying these conditions is the massive burden of Third World debt, which completely swamps attempts at genuine development, either human or economic. The Third World debt represents only 3% of assets for western banks (Logie, 1992), but it represents a crisis for the poorest countries in the world. Living standards in Latin America have not regained the level they were at before the colonial era, and it has been stated that industrialization has meant 'the modernization of poverty and little more' (Summerfield, 1989).

In the face of such a crisis, it is not surprising that long-term environmental and health concerns (such as cancer due to occupational and environmental exposures) take a back seat to the immediate struggle for survival. Poverty leads to population growth, air pollution, desertification and soil degradation (Smith & Stott, 1992) as well as to the maintenance or worsening of occupational health problems.

Alleviating poverty is not only a moral imperative but is also a prerequisite for environmental sustainability, and if the world is to survive resources must be shifted to the developing world (Smith & Stott, 1992). Currently, resources (and control of resources) are moving in the opposite direction (from poor to rich), as a result of debt repayment and structural adjustment programmes which produce increasing multinational penetration and reduced national sovereignty. In the context of Africa, Logie and Woodroffe (1993) therefore note that 'What is required is urgent debt relief, fairer terms of trade, more democratic government, and economic programmes which are designed by and for African people rather than the rich in the North.' The protection and improvement of health and the environment in developing countries and in the world as a whole will not be achieved by policies that continue to equate development with industrialization and that maintain or worsen existing inequalities in income, resources and power both within and between developing and industrialized countries.

References

Alubo, S.O. (1990) Debt crisis, health and health services in Africa. *Soc. Sci. Med.*, **31**, 639−648

Amasa, S.K. (1975) Arsenic pollution at Obuasi goldmine, town, and surrounding countryside. *Environ. Health Perspectives*, **12**, 131−135

Aniyam, C.A. (1989) The social costs of the International Monetary Fund's adjustment programs for poverty: the case of health care development in Ghana. *Int. J. Health Serv.*, **19**, 531−547

Anon. (1992) Let them eat pollution. *Economist*, **322** (7745), 82

Barry, M. (1991) The influence of the US tobacco industry on the health, economy, and environment of developing countries. *New Engl. J. Med.*, **324**, 917−920

Behrman, J.R. (1993) Health and economic growth: theory, evidence and policy. In: *Macroeconomic Environment and Health with Case Studies for Countries in Greatest Need*, Geneva, WHO, pp. 21−61

Bradshaw, E., McGlashan, N.D., Fitzgerald, D. & Harrington, J.S. (1982) Analyses of cancer incidence in black gold miners from southern Africa (1964−79). *Br. J. Cancer*, **46**, 737−748

Brown, E.R. (1976) Public health in imperialism: early Rockefeller programs at home and abroad. *Am. J. Public Health*, **66**, 897−903

Bullard, R.D. (1993) Reviewing the EPA's draft environmental equity report. *New Solutions*, **Spring**, 78−86

Bwititi, T., Chikuni, D., Loewenson, R., Murambiwa, W., Nhachi, C. & Nyazema, N. (1987) Health hazards in organophosphate use among farmworkers in the large scale farming sector. *Central Afr. Med. J.*, **33**, 120−125

Castleman, B. (1979) The export of hazardous factories to developing nations. *Int. J. Health Serv.*, **9**, 569−606

Castleman, B.I. (1985) The double standard in industrial hazards. In: Ives, J.H., ed., *The Export of Hazard*, London, Routledge & Kegan Paul, pp. 60−93

Castleman, B.I. & Purkavastha, P. (1985) The Bhopal disaster as a case study in double standards. In: Ives, J.H., ed., *The Export of Hazard*, London, Routledge & Kegan Paul, pp. 213−223

Chernomas, R. (1990) The debt-depression of the less developed world and public health. *Int. J. Health Serv.*, **20**, 537−543

Christiani, D.C. (1988) Modernization and occupational cancer. *J. Occup. Med.*, **30**, 975−976

Christiani, D.C., Durvasula, R. & Myers, J. (1990) Occupational health in developing countries: review of research needs. *Am. J. Ind. Med.*, **17**, 393−401

Cordova, A., Leal, G. & Martinez, C. (1986) Occupational health in Mexico: missing information. *Health Policy Planning*, **1**, 353−359

Cornia, G.A., Jolly, R. & Stewart, F. (1987) *Adjustment with a Human Face*, Oxford, Oxford University Press

Desowitz, R.S. (1976) How the wise men brought malaria to Africa. *Nat. Hist.*, 85

Doll, R. (1992) Health and the environment in the 1990s. *Am. J. Public Health*, **82**, 933−941

El Batawi, M.A. (1986) The Third Theodore F. Hatch symposium lecture. *Ann. Am. Conf. Gov. Ind. Hyg.*, **14**, 3−15

Elling, R.H. (1986) *The Struggle for Workers' Health. A Study of Six Industrialized Countries*, Amityville, NY, Baywood

Elling, R.H. (1988) Workers' health and safety (WHS) in cross-national perspective. *Am. J. Public Health*, **78**, 764−771

Engels, F. (1845) *The Condition of the Working Class in England*, London, Granada (1969 ed.), pp. 185−186

Esteva, G. (1992) Development. In: *The Development Dictionary*, London, Zed Press, pp. 6−24

Ferrer, A. & Cabral, R. (1991) Toxic epidemics caused by alimentary exposure to pesticides: a review. *Food Addit. Contam.*, **8**, 755−776

Forget, G. (1991) Pesticides in the third world. *J. Toxicol. Environ. Health*, **32**, 11−31

Hassan, A., Velasquez, E., Belmar, R., Coye, M., Drucker, E., Landrigan, P.J., Michaels, D. & Sidel, K.B. (1981) Mercury poisoning in Nicaragua: a case study of the export of environmental and occupational health hazards by a multinational corporation. *Int. J. Health Serv.*, **11**, 221−226

Huncharek, M. (1993) Exporting asbestos: disease and policy in the developing world. *J. Public Health Policy*, **14**, 51–65

Hunter, C. & Hughes, J. (1970) Disease and development in Africa. *Soc. Sci. Med.*, **3**, 443–485

Ives, J.H. (1985) The health effects of the transfer of technology to the developing world: report and case studies. In: Ives, J.H., ed., *The Export of Hazard*, London, Routledge & Kegan Paul, pp. 172–191

Jeyaratnam, J. (1985) 1984 and occupational health in developing countries. *Scand. J. Work Environ. Health*, **11**, 229–234

Kanji, N., Kanji, N. & Manji, F. (1991) From development to sustained crisis: structural adjustment, equity and health. *Soc. Sci. Med.*, **33**, 985–993

Kasperson, J.X. & Kasperson, R.E. (1987) Priorities in profile: managing risks in developing countries. *Risk Abstr.*, **4**, 113–118

Kloos, H. (1982) Development, drought and famine in the Awash Valley of Ethiopia. *Afr. Stud. Rev.*, **22**, 21–48

Kloos, H., Desole, G. & Lemma, A. (1981) Intestinal parasitism in seminomadic pastoralists and subsistence farmers in and around irrigation schemes in Ethiopia. *Soc. Sci. Med.*, **15B**, 457–469

Landrigan, P.J. (1992) Commentary: environmental disease—a preventable epidemic. *Am. J. Public Health*, **82**, 941–943

Lanoix, J. (1958) Relation between irrigation engineering and bilharzia. *World Health Org. Bull.*, **8**, 1101

Laurel, A. (1981) Mortality and working conditions in agriculture in underdeveloped countries. *Int. J. Health Services*, **11**, 3–20

Loewenson, R. (1988) Labour insecurity and health: an epidemiological study in Zimbabwe. *Soc. Sci. Med.*, **27**, 733–741

Loewenson, R. (1991) Workers' activities in Zimbabwe. *Afr. Newslett. Occup. Health Saf.*, **1**, 88–89

Loewenson, R. (1993) Socioeconomic trends and health in developing countries. In: *Proceedings of the NIVA Course on Occupational Health Research in Developing Countries, Stockholm, 24–28 May 1993* (in press)

Logie, D. (1992) The great exterminator of children. *Br. Med. J.*, **304**, 1423–1246

Logie, D.E. & Woodroffe, J. (1993) Structural adjustment: the wrong prescription for Africa? *Br. Med. J.*, **307**, 41–44

Lukindo, J.K. (1993) Comprehensive survey of the informal section in Tanzania. *Afr. Newslett. Occup. Health Saf.*, **3**, 36–37

Mandal, G. & Gosh, M. (1976) *Economics of the Green Revolution*, Bombay, Asia Publishing House

Marmot, M.G. & McDowell, M.E. (1986) Mortality decline and widening social inequalities. *Lancet*, **ii**, 274–276

Matte, T.D., Figureueroa, J.P., Ostrowski, S., Burr, G., Flesch, J.P., Keenlyside, R.A. & Baker, E.L. (1989) Lead poisoning among household members exposed to lead–acid battery repair shops in Kingston, Jamaica. *Int. J. Epidemiol.*, **18**, 874–881

Mazuri, A. (1986) *The Africans: A Triple Heritage*, New York, Little Brown

McConnell, R., Cordon, M., Murray, D.L. & Magnotti, R. (1992) Hazards of closed pesticide mixing and loading systems: the paradox of protective technology in the Third World. *Br. J. Ind. Med.*, **49**, 615–619

McCord, C. & Freeman, H.P. (1990) Excess mortality in Harlem. *New Engl. J. Med.*, **322**, 173–177

McKeown, T. (1988) *The Origins of Human Disease*, Oxford, Basil Blackwell

McMichael, A.J. (1993) Global environmental change and human population health: a conceptual and scientific challenge for epidemiology. *Int. J. Epidemiol.*, **22**, 1–8

Michaels, D., Barrera, C. & Gacharra, M.G. (1985) Economic development and occupational health in Latin America. *Am. J. Public Health*, **75**, 536–542

Navarro, V. (1984) Policies on exportation of hazardous substances in western developed countries. *New Engl. J. Med.*, **311**, 546–548

Noweir, M.H. (1986) Occupational health in developing countries with special reference to Egypt. *Am. J. Ind. Med.*, **9**, 125–141

Ong, C.N., Jeyaratnam, J. & Koh, D. (1993) Factors influencing the assessment and control of occupational hazards in developing countries. *Environ. Res.*, **60**, 112–123

Onimode, B., ed. (1989) *The IMF, the World Bank and the African Debt*, Vols 1 and 2, London, Zed Press

Packard, R.M. (1989) Industrial production, health and disease in sub-Saharan Africa. *Soc. Sci. Med.*, **28**, 475–496

Pappas, G., Queen, S., Hadden, W. & Fisher, G. (1993) The increasing disparity in mortality between socioeconomic groups in the United States, 1960 and 1986. *New Engl. J. Med.*, **329**, 103–109

Pearce, N.E., Marshall, S. & Borman, B. (1991) Undiminished social class differences in New Zealand men. *N.Z. Med. J.*, **104**, 153–156

Pinstrup–Andersen, P. (1993) Economic crises and policy reforms during the 1980s and their impact on the poor. In: *Macroeconomic Environment and Health with Case Studies for Countries in Greatest Need*, Geneva, WHO, pp. 85–115

Pomare, E. & de Boer, G. (1988) *Hauora: Maori Standards of Health, 1970–1984*, Wellington, Department of Health

Quinn, M.M., Punnett, L., Christiani, D.C., Levenstein, C. & Wegman, D.H. (1987) Modernization and trends in occupational health and safety in the People's Republic of China 1981–1986. *Am. J. Ind. Med.*, **12**, 499–506

Roemer, M.I. & Roemer, R. (1990) Global health, national development, and the role of government. *Am. J. Public Health*, **80**, 1188–1192

Sachs, W. (1990) On the archaeology of the development idea. *Ecologist*, **20**, 42–43

Sen, A. (1988) *Levels of Poverty: Policy and Change* (World Bank Staff Working Paper No. 401), Washington DC, World Bank

Simonato, L. (1986) Aspects of occupational cancer in developing countries. In: Khogali, M., Omar, Y.T., Gjorgov, A. & Ismail, A.S., eds, *Proceedings of the 2nd UICC Conference on Cancer Prevention, Kuwait, 1984*, Oxford, Pergamon Press, pp. 101–106

Smith, C. & Beckman, S.L. (1991) *Export of Pesticides from US Ports in 1990*, Los Angeles, Foundation for Advancement in Science and Education

Smith, R. & Stott, R. (1992) A meeting of rich and poor. *Br. Med. J.*, **304**, 1392–1393

Spence, D.P.S., Hotchkiss, J., Wiliams, C.S.D & Davies, P.D.O. (1993) Tuberculosis and poverty. *Br. Med. J.*, **307**, 759–761

Steinmetz, K.A. & Potter, J.D. (1991) Vegetables, fruit and cancer: I. Epidemiology. *Cancer Causes Control*, **2**, 325–357

Stewart, F. (1991) The many faces of adjustment. *World Dev.*, **19**, 1847–1864

Summerfield, D. (1989) Western economics and third world health. *Lancet*, **ii**, 551–552

Taba, A.-H. (1981) Problems of occupational carcinogenesis in developing countries. *Cancer Detect. Prev.*, **4**, 25–30

Taussig, M. (1978) Nutrition, development and foreign aid. *Int. J. Health Serv.*, **8**, 101–121

Testa Tambellini, A. (1993) Occupational and environmental health in South America: the result of rapid changes in social and economic conditions. In: *Proceedings of the 24th Congress of the International Commission on Occupational Health, Nice, September 26–30 1993*, pp. 153–157

Tolba, M.K. & El-Kholy, O.A., eds (1992) *The World Environment, 1972–1992: Two Decades of Challenge*, London, Chapman & Hall

Tomatis, L. (1992) Poverty and cancer. *Cancer Epidemiol. Biomarkers Prev.*, **1**, 167–175

Tomatis, L., Aitio, A., Day, N.E., Heseltine, E., Kaldor, J., Miller, A.B., Parkin, D.M. & Riboli, E., eds (1990) *Cancer: Causes, Occurrence and Control* (IARC Scientific Publications No. 100), Lyon, IARC, p. 216

Victoria, C. & Blank, N. (1980) Epidemiology of infant mortality in Rio Grande do Sul, Brazil. *J. Trop. Med. Hyg.*, **83**, 177–186

Visagie, M.E., Du-Plessis, J.P., Groothof, G., Alberts, A. & Laubscher, N.F. (1974) Changes in vitamin A and C levels in black mine-workers. *S. Afr. Med. J.*, **48**, 2502–2506

WHO (1981) *Recommended Health-based Limits in Occupational Exposure to Selected Organic Solvents. Report of a WHO Study Group* (Technical Report Series 664), Geneva

WHO (1983) *Apartheid and Health*, Geneva

WHO (1992) *Our Planet, Our Health: Report of the WHO Commission on Health and Environment*, Geneva

Wilkinson, R. (1992) National mortality rates: the impact of inequality. *Am. J. Public Health*, **82**, 1082–1084

Wimberley, D.W. (1990) Investment dependence and alternative explanations of third world mortality: a cross-national study. *Am. Sociol. Rev.*, **55**, 75–91

Wisner, B. (1980) Nutritional consequences of the articulation of capitalist and non-capitalist modes of production in eastern Kenya. *Rural Afr.*, **9**, 99–132

World Bank (1989) *Sub-Saharan Africa: From Crisis to Sustainable Growth*, Washington DC

Zengeya, S., Sena, A., Zanza, J., Loewenson, R. & Laing, R. (1982) The health status of mineworkers communities in Zimbabwe. *Cent. Afr. Med. J.*, **28**, 15–159

Chapter 2. Transfer of Hazardous Industries

J. Jeyaratnam

The transfer of hazardous industries to the developing world is of current and growing concern. The main factors that lead to such transfer are stringent domestic, industrial and environmental regulations and increasing labour costs in the industrialized world and several factors in developing countries such as cheap labour, unemployment, national drives towards industrialization and lack of (or poor implementation of) labour, environmental and industrial regulations (Jeyaratnam, 1990). The siting of industrial plants can result in serious problems for the local community if workers are not properly trained or are unaware of the technological requirements of the job. Poor or careless safety measures and plant management by the originating company can also contribute to devastation of the community. Such a situation occurred in Bhopal, India, in late 1984 in the Union Carbide plant manufacturing methyl isocyanate (LaDou, 1991).

Moreover, the standards established for exposure to chemicals are not uniform among countries and considerations are not usually health-based but are tempered by economic, social, educational, employment and other concerns. In many developing countries, exposure standards are often nonexistent, not enforced or too lax to be of actual preventive use. As a consequence, control of industrial hazards is in practice different for industrialized and developing countries (Jeyaratnam, 1990).

Factors that contribute to transfer

In industrialized countries, stringent regulations and controls for safety and health have made it more expensive for industries to operate. In addition, labour costs have increased markedly. Arguably the most compelling reason for taking hazardous industries out of industrialized countries, however, is an increasing awareness among the general public about the health consequences of industries and their waste products — 'the green movement' — which has resulted in a strong lobby for the safety of the environment and its impact on human health.

Several factors in the developing world tend to attract hazardous materials and industries. A strong economic consideration, particularly a desperate need for 'hard' currency, motivates many countries. Further, a cheap labour force, lack of legislation and poor implementation of such legislation make the countries of the developing world attractive for relocating hazardous industries. Most countries of the developing world are pursuing a path of rapid industrialization and are willing to take anything and everything offered, however hazardous.

Examples of transfer of hazardous materials and industries

The transfer of hazardous industries was described by Castleman (1980) as 'double standards', in that hazardous industrial processes are set up in one country to serve markets in another country where those processes would not be allowed to function. He lists a number of such cases, as shown in Table 1. Several examples are discussed in more detail below.

Table 1. Examples of transfer of hazardous industries

Industry	Foreign involvement	Location	Type of hazard or risk reported
Asbestos milling	Subsidiary mining operation	South Africa	Severe asbestosis in children
α-Naphthylamine manufacture	Not known	Outside the United Kingdom	Bladder cancer
Benzidine dye manufacture		Outside the United Kingdom	Bladder cancer
Asbestos textile manufacture	Subsidiary	Agua Prieta and Juarez, Mexico	Workers not informed or provided with clothing change, neighbourhood pollution
Asbestos friction product and textile manufacture	74% ownership	Bombay, India	Numerous uncontrolled hazards, workers not informed or given findings of medical examinations
Asbestos		Countries without existing requirements	No warning labels
Asbestos–cement manufacture	Minority ownership, exclusive marketing of exports, raw material sales, plant design and construction supervision	Ahmedabad, India	Water pollution, solid waste dumping, no warnings on products
Asbestos brake lining manufacture	25% ownership	Madras, India	Solid waste dumping
Asbestos brake shoe manufacture		Republic of Korea	Substandard working conditions
Asbestos textiles	Subsidiary	South Africa	
Asbestos milling	Subsidiary	Quebec, Canada	No controls on workplace dust
Asbestos brake shoes	Subsidiary	Cork, Ireland	Newly built plant using asbestos as raw material
Epoxy spraying		Shipyards outside Denmark	Eczema, cancer (?)

Table 1 (contd)

Industry reported	Foreign involvement	Location	Type of hazard or risk re-
Chromate and di-chromate manu-facture	Partial ownership	Lecheria, Mexico	Waste dumping, workplace exposures resulted in nasal septum perforation
Dye manufacture	Partial ownership	Bombay, India	Water pollution
Mercury cell chlorine plant	40% ownership and management of the plant	Managua, Nicaragua	Mercury poisoning, water pollution
Steelmaking	Minority ownership and plant design	Malaysia	Air pollution, workplace hazards
Polyvinyl chloride	Partial ownership	Malaysia	High exposure to vinyl chloride manufacture
Arsenical pesti-cides manufacture	Subsidiary	Malaysia	Symptoms of arsenic poisoning in workers, no monitoring of exposure

Adapted from Castleman (1983)

Hazardous waste

The transfer of hazardous waste from the industrialized countries to the countries of the developing world is also an area of major concern. Western European countries produce between 30 and 40 million tonnes of hazardous waste annually, while the USA produces more than 200 million tonnes and Japan, 700 000 tonnes. These data are not readily comparable, however, as the USA, for instance, defines 450 materials as hazardous, Germany, 85 and Japan, a mere 8 as hazardous out of 23 000 compounds in use. There are no reliable figures for the volume of hazardous waste exported, but the US Environmental Protection Agency has estimated that illegal shipments outnumber legal ones by 8:1 (LaDou, 1991).

Africa has become the prime target for dumping toxic waste (Smith & George, 1988). For example, as environmental laws in western Europe dictate that polychlorinated biphenyls be incinerated at high temperatures, it costs more than US$ 2000 per tonne to dispose of this type of chemical waste; however, an Italian company was able to persuade a Nigerian to accept 2500 tonnes of polychlorinated biphenyl waste on his land for a service fee of US$ 100 per month. The company that arranged for the disposal may make US$ 2.5 million on this arrangement (LaDou, 1991). Vir (1988) identified several other African nations, such as Guinea, Benin, Ethiopia, Guinea-Bissau, Sierra Leone and the Gambia, which have faced similar problems relating to toxic wastes. For instance, small countries such as Guinea-Bissau have been offered up to four times their gross national product in exchange for receiving 15 million tonnes of European toxic materials (LaDou, 1991).

It is in this context of enormous potential commercial gain that the legislative efforts to control the traffic in hazardous wastes should be considered. The toughest legislative proposals have come from the 16 West African countries grouped under the Economic Community of West African States, which have agreed to make it a criminal offence to facilitate the dumping of toxic waste. The Organization of African Unity has adopted the African Convention on the Ban on Imports of All Forms of Hazardous Wastes into Africa, and the Basel Convention on the Control of Transboundary Movement of Hazardous Wastes and their Disposal (see Chapter 10) was adopted by 116 countries and the European Community in 1989 (Tolba & El-Kholy, 1992). Despite the good intentions of the African and similar proposals, substantial problems still exist in the definition, legal drafting and enforcement of environmental legislation (Smith & George, 1988).

Banned pesticides

The transfer of banned pesticides has existed for several decades. The pesticide leptophos, which could not be sold in the USA as it was not registered with the US Environmental Protection Agency, was manufactured in the USA exclusively for foreign markets; a single company exported this pesticide to more than 30 different nations, including Egypt, where it was reported that its use had resulted in death and illness in many farmers and the deaths of over 1000 water buffalo (Agege, 1985). Pesticides such as aldrin, dieldrin, heptachlor and chlordane are also banned in the USA but are made available for export (Smith & Beckman, 1991).

Most pesticides produced in developing countries are manufactured by foreign-owned companies or local companies with capital invested by foreigners. Many newly industrialized countries manufacture increased quantities of pesticides that are banned in developed countries. DDT is a compelling example: It has been illegal to produce or use DDT in the USA and Europe since the 1970s, but it is entirely legal for US and European companies to manufacture DDT in other countries that do not ban its production, and its worldwide production is at record levels.

Asbestos

The best example of the flight of hazardous industries is the manufacture of asbestos products (Brenan & Lucas, 1983). The carcinogenic potential of asbestos has been established for many years, and controls on the manufacture of asbestos products have been tightened in almost every industrialized nation.   The manufacture of asbestos-based products has, however, shifted to countries such as Brazil, India, Pakistan, Indonesia and the Republic of Korea. For example, Johannig et al. (1991) reported the transfer of Rex Industrie Produkte, a German asbestos textile plant, to Pusan, Republic of Korea, thereby evading the German health and safety standards and requirements. Such asbestos products are often re-imported: Germany and the USA are among the biggest importers of asbestos products from the Republic of Korea. Despite the occupational and environmental hazards posed by asbestos products, Canada promotes asbestos in the Third World, where demand for low-cost building materials outweighs health concerns (LaDou, 1991). Canadian exports of asbestos to the Republic of Korea increased to 44 000 tonnes in 1989 from 5000 tonnes in 1980; exports to Pakistan climbed to 6000 tonnes from 300 tonnes over the same period. Canada now exports close to half its asbestos to the Third World (Dahl, 1989).

Lead

A case report from Taiwan (Wang *et al.*, 1992) indicates another potential source of contamination in the developing world. A battery recycling plant in Taipei, China, imports large amounts of waste batteries from the USA and Japan to extract lead. As a consequence, a worker was admitted to the National Taiwan University Hospital as an overt case of lead poisoning with anaemia and bilateral peripheral neuropathy. The investigators observed that the factory was also a source of environmental pollution, resulting in higher than average levels of lead in air, and that a kindergarten school was located in its immediate vicinity.

Other examples

Japan is also beginning to site its industrial plants in South-East Asian nations. In collaboration with a Japanese company, companies were set up in Malaysia to extract rare earth chlorides from monazite. The monazite in Malaysia contains 7% thorium, a radioactive element with a half-life of one billion years; the radiation level was reported to be 800 times the background level, and even after attempts at enclosure the radioactivity was still 150 times background (Hidaka, 1987). Recently, after a seven-year legal battle by residents and environmentalists against Asian Rare Earth, a company owned by Japan's Mitsubishi Kasei Corporation, the Malaysian operation was closed by a ruling of the High Court in Malaysia; however, the ruling was subsequently reversed by a High Court decision.

US industries have recently developed a silent contract with the Mexican Government which in large measure waives responsibility for the safe use of industrial toxic materials and their waste disposal. 'Maquiladoras' are manufacturing facilities in Mexico in which workers earn much lower wages than workers in plants on the US side of the border (LaDou, 1991). Similar facilities are being opened by Japanese, Canadian and German companies. Juarez, a Mexican city, already has 300 such plants and has almost doubled its population; yet Juarez has no sewage-treatment system or hazardous waste-disposal facilities that would meet US standards (Cordes *et al.*, 1989).

International controls

Any control mechanism must be considered in the context of moral issues and the fact that such sales and transfers are often largely for commercial reasons (Jeyaratnam, 1990). UNEP has as one of its objectives the establishment of a warning system for countries in which the environment and human health may be affected by the export of hazardous substances. The London Guidelines for the Exchange of Information on Chemicals in International Trade (UNEP, 1989) is an example of its activity. One of its general principles is that both states of export and states of import should protect human health and the environment against potential harm by exchanging information on chemicals in international trade. One of the mechanisms for control is the procedure of obtaining prior informed consent. The International Register of Potentially Toxic Chemicals identifies all chemicals banned or severely restricted by five or more countries.

The Organisation for Economic Co-operation and Development has advocated the 'polluter pays' principle and, in cooperation with the United Nations and the European

Economic Community, has been able to restrict the manufacture and use of certain chemicals in all 24 of its Member States (Seferovich, 1981). Legislative control to reduce the hazard resulting from the transfer and export of banned chemicals and industries differs from controls necessary for the protection of, say, the ozone layer. In the latter case, many countries are capable of producing the chemicals that damage the ozone layer; in the former case, only the countries where the banned substances are manufactured have the potential to do harm, if they do not export them.

In the past, the health effects of hazardous industries were considered to be a problem restricted to workers and to people in the immediate vicinity of the industry. These effects are, however, becoming recognized increasingly as not a local but a global problem (Jeyaratnam, 1990). One aspect of global involvement is re-importation. For instance, in the USA, the US Environmental Protection Agency is responsible for setting maximal levels of pesticide residues allowed in imported foods; however, a spot check showed that 10% of shipments contained residues of unregistered or severely restricted pesticides (Vagliano, 1981). Chemicals such as aldrin, dieldrin, heptachlor and chlordane that are banned in the USA but made available for export have been re-imported as contaminants of cocoa from Ecuador, coffee from Costa Rica and sugar and tea from India (Seferovich, 1981).

From the standpoint of international law, the decision in the Trail Smelter Arbitration case is significant (Seferovich, 1981). In that arbitration, emission of sulfur dioxide fumes from a private smelting company operating in British Columbia, Canada, caused harm to timber and crops in Washington State, USA. An international tribunal held Canada liable under international law for the act of its nationals.

Concluding remarks

There is no justification for the sale or transfer of materials banned in one country, on the basis of their harmful effects on human health, to another country for commercial reasons. An argument often stated in justification of such transfer of banned materials and industries is that each nation has the right to decide for itself its own needs and requirements. That position implies that the donor country has no responsibility or right to decide what it exports.

A parallel can be drawn with the sale of arms: There is global agreement that nuclear weapons and other military equipment are sold or transferred at the discretion of the manufacturing nation, and not merely at the request of the purchasing nation. The manufacturing nation assumes responsibility to contain the proliferation of agents that are likely to damage mankind. The Bush administration in the USA, in an effort to keep developing nations from building chemical and biological arsenals, was prepared to restrict US exports of commonly used chemicals and manufacturing equipment that can also be used to make weapons (Auerbach, 1991). That effort goes further than current controls exerted by the loosely knit group of 23 countries known as the Australia Group to halt the spread of chemical and biological weapons (Jeyaratnam, 1990). A similar approach could be taken for chemicals and industries that are banned in developed countries for reasons of their adverse effects on human health and their potential to damage the global environment.

References

Agege, C.O. (1985) Dumping of dangerous American products overseas: should Congress sit and watch. *J. World Trade Law*, **19**, 403–410

Auerbach, S. (1991) US to curb exports of chemicals that can be used for arms. *Int. Herald Tribune*, **28 February**

Brenan, T.A. & Lucas, W.J. (1983) Legal strategy for controlling the export of hazardous industries to developing countries: the case of asbestos. *Yale J. Public Order*, **9**, 275–314

Castleman, B.J. (1980) The 'double standards' in industrial hazards. *Public Health Rev.*, **9**, 169–184

Castleman, B.J. (1983) The double standards in industrial hazards. *Int. J. Health Serv.*, **13**, 5–14

Cordes, D.H., Ra, B.F., Schwartz, I. & Rea, J. (1989) Mexico, macquiladoras and occupational medicine. *Asia–Pacific J. Public Health*, **3**, 61–67

Dahl, J. (1989) Canada encourages mining of asbestos, sells to the Third World. *Wall Street J.*, **12 September**

Hidaka, J. (1987) Mitsubishi subsidiary faces battle over radioactive pollution in Malaysia. *Japan Times*, **9 January**

Jeyaratnam, J. (1990) The transfer of hazardous industries. *J. Soc. Occup. Med.*, **40**, 123–126

Johannig, E., Selikoff, I.J. & Goldberg, M. (1991) *Asbestos Health Hazard Evaluation in South Korea. Asbestos Textile Manufacturing*, New York, Mount Sinai Medical Center

LaDou, J. (1991) The export of industrial hazards to developing countries. In: Jeyaratnam, J., ed., *Occupational Health in Developing Countries*, Oxford, Oxford University Press, pp. 340–358

Seferovich, P.B. (1981) United States export of banned products: legal and moral implications. *Denver J. Int. Law Policy*, **10**, 537–560

Smith, C. & Beckman, S.L. (1991) *Export of Pesticides from US Ports in 1990*, Los Angeles, Foundation for Advancement in Science and Education

Smith, P. & George, A. (1988) The dumping grounds. *South*, **August**, 37–39

Tolba, M.K. & El-Kholy, O.A., eds (1992) *The World Environment 1972–1992: Two Decades of Challenge*, London, Chapman & Hall

UNEP (1989) *London Guidelines for the Exchange of Information on Chemicals in International Trade*, Nairobi

Vagliano, B. (1981) Any place but here: A critique of United States hazardous export policy. *Brooklyn J. Int. Law*, VII, 329–363

Vir, A.K. (1988) Africa says no to toxic dumping schemes. *Environ. Action*, **November/December**, 26–28

Wang, J.D., Jang, C.S., Hwang, J.Y. & Chen, Z.S. (1992) Lead contamination around a kindergarten near a battery recycling plant. *Bull. Environ. Contam. Toxicol.*, **49**, 23–30

Chapter 3. Burden of Cancer in Developing Countries

P. Pisani

This chapter gives an overview of the incidence of occupationally related cancers in developing countries. The 11 cancer sites that were selected for the analysis are those that have been linked most consistently to occupational exposures in developed countries and for which estimates of worldwide incidence and mortality are available. They are: oral cavity (ICD-9 140−149), larynx (161), lung (162), oesophagus (150), stomach (151), liver (155), pancreas (157), urinary bladder (188), kidney (189), all lymphomas (200−203), including multiple myeloma, and all leukaemias (204−208). Although non-occupational factors (e.g. cigarette smoking) are the major causes of many of these cancers (e.g. lung), occupational factors may still play a significant role.

The estimates presented are derived from the results of Parkin *et al.* (1993) and Pisani *et al.* (1993), and the methods of estimation used are described in detail in the original papers. Nevertheless, it should be noted that the amount and quality of data available vary enormously, and the paucity of data from developing countries is striking. In particular, no attempt was made to estimate the occurrence of some cancers at specific sites, such as non-melanoma skin cancer or pleural mesothelioma, for which the reporting is subject to high error rates.

For the purpose of this analysis, 10 geographical regions were determined: five covering developing regions—Africa, China, Asia (excluding China and Japan), Melanesia/Polynesia and Latin America (comprising Central and South America and the Caribbean); and five constituting the more developed regions of the world—North America, Europe, Australia/New Zealand, Japan and the former USSR. China is represented as a single region as it accounts for 22% of the world population.

Estimated incidences of occupation-related cancers in developing countries

Infectious and reproductive diseases and malnutrition are still the main health priorities for developing countries. Nevertheless, a substantial part of the difference in cancer risk between industrialized countries and the rest of the world is due to the young age distribution in the less developed regions, where, in 1985, 37% of the population was under the age of 15 compared to 22% reported for developed countries.

Table 1 shows age-standardized cancer incidence rates for men and women by region and cancer site. Overall cancer incidence in men is 1.8 times higher in developed countries than in developing countries; the rates are higher for most of the specific cancers considered except for cancers of the mouth/pharynx, oesophagus and liver. The rate ratios vary from 4.0 for kidney cancer to 1.2 for stomach cancer; those for oesophageal and liver cancers are 0.5 and that for oral cancer is 0.8. In women, the pattern is similar, but the rate ratios are lower: 1.3 for all sites, 2.8 for kidney cancer (again, the highest observed)

31

Table 1. Annual age-standardized incidence rates per 100 000 for cancers at 11 selected sites and all sites around 1985, by geographic region

Region	Oral cavity	Oesophagus	Stomach	Liver	Pancreas	Larynx	Lung	Urinary bladder	Kidney	Lymphoma	Leukaemia	All sites
Males												
Africa	11.65	9.87	9.70	16.42	2.03	5.55	9.83	10.34	1.49	11.21	2.42	144.05
China	8.71	22.14	43.14	21.83	5.98	2.76	28.31	6.07	2.11	5.90	5.92	189.60
Asia, other	21.08	7.47	9.66	7.39	1.53	7.22	18.46	4.01	1.32	5.31	3.22	119.65
Polynesia/Micronesia	9.99	3.42	9.41	8.46	4.05	3.81	34.79	3.48	1.53	4.88	8.03	135.92
Latin America	13.43	8.96	30.32	3.34	4.74	8.75	29.21	9.54	3.59	10.39	5.78	216.27
Northern America	14.16	4.94	8.77	2.86	8.69	7.50	73.55	23.05	10.39	19.40	10.13	342.89
Former USSR	15.68	9.16	44.04	5.20	6.88	9.05	63.98	8.39	4.25	5.91	6.51	223.11
Europe	12.09	5.51	21.39	5.72	7.51	8.84	58.54	17.25	7.97	12.16	7.62	269.01
Japan	4.47	8.86	74.79	22.94	9.14	3.25	35.80	6.86	4.35	7.41	5.68	238.30
Australia/New Zealand	15.08	4.55	13.02	2.20	7.23	5.21	53.03	16.15	7.91	16.17	9.64	294.45
Developing countries	14.94	13.04	23.65	13.01	3.49	5.64	22.15	6.04	1.87	6.81	4.21	157.43
Developed countries	12.46	6.36	28.31	6.80	7.87	7.96	60.82	2.64	7.45	12.23	7.89	276.51
Age-standardized rate ratio	0.8	0.5	1.2	0.5	2.2	1.4	2.8	2.6	4.0	1.8	1.9	1.8
Females												
Africa	6.98	3.84	7.25	6.85	1.61	0.80	2.67	3.25	1.39	6.40	1.96	147.02
China	5.98	12.14	19.36	9.05	5.94	1.13	12.15	2.67	1.72	4.23	4.42	158.58
Asia, other	12.57	5.16	5.60	3.28	1.08	1.32	4.60	1.13	0.78	3.52	2.53	124.38
Polynesia/Micronesia	4.55	0.78	5.22	2.63	1.80	0.44	10.83	0.75	1.25	3.05	5.27	120.33
Latin America	3.83	2.76	15.09	2.55	3.12	1.13	7.45	2.38	1.90	7.53	4.34	206.06
Northern America	5.07	1.37	4.23	1.33	6.17	1.26	28.87	6.15	5.17	13.70	6.83	277.55
Former USSR	3.05	3.01	19.45	2.51	3.51	0.37	7.71	1.16	2.19	3.74	4.64	130.80
Europe	2.76	1.28	10.59	2.77	4.89	0.66	9.84	3.67	4.19	8.07	5.19	204.02
Japan	1.82	1.50	35.16	6.44	5.19	0.23	10.28	1.92	1.63	4.22	3.76	154.20
Australia/New Zealand	4.81	2.32	5.90	0.76	5.14	0.58	14.49	4.74	4.46	11.61	6.16	238.02
Developing countries	8.63	7.23	11.74	5.63	3.10	1.17	7.35	2.08	1.32	4.61	3.20	148.98
Developed countries	3.25	1.74	13.73	2.73	4.87	0.66	13.30	3.44	3.67	7.91	5.30	197.63
Age-standardized rate ratio	0.4	0.2	1.2	0.5	1.6	0.6	1.8	1.7	2.8	1.7	1.7	1.3

and 0.2 for cancer of the oesophagus; cancer of the larynx is less frequent in women in industrialized countries, but it is very rare in this sex everywhere.

Of the 7.6 million new cases of cancer occurring each year in the world, 4 million occur in developing countries, and the overall incidence is slightly higher in males than in females: 3 849 400 *versus* 3 774 200, respectively (Table 2). In developing countries, the 11 cancer sites considered accounted for 72.1% of all cancers in males and 36.7% in females (Table 3). This striking difference is due to the predominant importance of cancers of the cervix and breast in women (not related to occupation and therefore not included in the analysis), coupled with the increasing incidence of tobacco-related cancers in men (included in this analysis).

Of the 11 sites chosen, the most frequent cancer in males living in developing countries is that of the stomach (this was also the commonest cause of death from cancer in developed countries until 30 years ago), accounting for 14.2% of neoplasms in males and 7.5% in females. Lung cancer follows closely (13.2%). The frequency of cancer of the oral cavity and pharynx was very high in both males and females, being the third commonest cancer in males and the second commonest in females. In Asian countries (excluding China), it accounted for 17% of all cancers in males. As the component subsites of this group have different relative frequencies by region, the grouping makes international comparisons difficult. In South-East Asia, most such cases are cancers of the tongue and gum, which can be attributed to the popular habit of chewing tobacco and other cured vegetables. In China, the nasopharynx is the most frequent subsite of cancer; its occurrence is attributed to genetic predisposition and to a variety of environmental factors, including exposure to fumes and dusts. Oral cancer is less common in industrialized countries, especially among women, and is largely attributed to alcohol consumption and tobacco smoking. Oesophageal cancer accounts for 7.7% of all cancers in males and 4.5% in females in developing countries, compared to 2.3% and 1.0%, respectively, in developed regions. Liver cancer is very rare in developed countries, with the single exception of Japan, where the age-standardized rate of 22.9 is the highest reported in men. The other regions of high risk are China (21.8 in males and 19.4 in females) and Africa (16.4 in males and 6.8 in females). Most of the cases in developing countries are attributed to infection with hepatitis B and C viruses.

Cancers of the lung, larynx, bladder, pancreas and kidney are more consistently related to tobacco smoking, and their incidence is definitely higher in industrialized regions. Lung cancer was by far the most frequent cancer in the world for males in 1985, with a total estimated number of 677 000 new cases per year, 39% of which occurred in developing countries (Parkin *et al.*, 1993). It is 3.7 times less frequent among women.

Lymphomas and leukaemias are heterogeneous groups of morphological entities characterized by different descriptive epidemiology, but estimates for subtypes could not be attempted because in many instances the source data were available only in grouped form. The risk for lymphomas has been increasing over the last 30 years in industrialized countries (Devesa & Fears, 1992), which have the highest rates in the world; the rate ratio of developed to developing countries is 1.8 in men and 1.7 in women. It is remarkable that the high incidence rate estimated for Africa is very close to that reported for Europe.

Table 2. Estimated numbers (thousands) of new cases of cancer in 1985, by geographical region and site

Region	Oral cavity	Oesophagus	Stomach	Liver	Pancreas	Larynx	Lung	Urinary bladder	Kidney	Lymphoma/multiple myeloma	Leukaemia	All sites
Males												
Africa	16.7	13.4	13.4	26.0	2.9	7.3	13.0	13.6	2.8	21.3	4.7	211.7
China	37.9	89.3	176.3	96.9	25.7	11.6	115.4	25.5	9.4	28.5	30.7	815.5
Asia, other	113.9	38.7	51.5	40.7	8.0	37.4	95.9	20.4	7.9	34.8	24.4	661.1
Polynesia/Micronesia	0.0	0.0	0.0	0.0	0.0	0.0	0.1	0.0	0.0	0.0	0.0	0.4
Latin America	17.6	11.3	38.6	4.4	6.0	11.1	37.0	11.9	4.9	15.7	10.2	286.6
Northern America	21.4	7.7	14.1	4.5	14.1	11.5	116.7	37.4	16.0	29.7	15.5	547.7
Former USSR	20.0	11.2	54.2	6.4	8.4	11.7	79.6	9.9	5.4	7.6	8.2	277.4
Europe	36.6	17.3	69.1	18.3	24.1	27.1	187.0	56.2	24.5	36.2	22.0	845.1
Japan	3.2	6.4	53.8	16.5	6.6	2.3	25.9	4.9	3.1	5.2	3.6	170.3
Australia/New Zealand	1.6	0.5	1.4	0.2	0.8	0.6	5.8	1.8	0.8	1.7	1.0	32.0
Developing countries	186.8	152.8	279.8	168.2	42.6	67.3	261.4	71.5	24.9	100.5	70.1	1977.3
Developed countries	82.8	43.1	192.7	45.9	54.0	53.1	415.1	110.2	49.8	80.4	50.3	1872.4
Females												
Africa	11.2	5.8	11.3	11.6	2.5	1.2	4.0	5.1	2.9	12.9	4.0	247.0
China	26.7	52.4	84.8	40.6	25.8	4.8	53.1	11.6	7.6	19.3	21.6	707.8
Asia, other	69.7	27.8	30.5	18.0	5.7	7.1	24.6	5.9	4.9	21.6	18.6	721.9
Polynesia/Micronesia	0.0	0.0	0.0	0.0	0.0	0.0	0.0	0.0	0.0	0.0	0.0	0.3
Latin America	5.6	3.9	21.7	3.7	4.4	1.6	10.6	3.4	3.1	11.9	7.9	308.0
Northern America	9.4	2.8	9.2	2.6	13.6	2.4	55.9	13.1	9.8	26.1	12.7	527.7
Former USSR	6.7	7.1	44.2	5.7	8.3	0.8	17.5	2.8	4.6	6.8	8.4	274.5
Europe	11.0	5.9	48.6	12.3	22.6	2.6	42.0	16.9	16.8	31.3	18.8	823.7
Japan	1.6	1.5	31.2	6.0	4.9	0.2	9.7	1.9	1.4	3.7	2.7	132.4
Australia/New Zealand	0.6	0.3	0.8	0.1	0.7	0.1	1.9	0.6	0.6	1.5	0.7	29.0
Developing countries	113.5	89.9	148.3	73.9	38.4	14.7	92.4	26.0	18.5	65.8	52.2	1987.2
Developed countries	29.3	17.7	134.0	26.8	50.1	6.0	126.9	35.4	33.3	69.4	43.3	1787.3

Table 3. Percentage of total cancers in the different regions by site

Region	Oral cavity	Oesophagus	Stomach	Liver	Pancreas	Larynx	Lung	Urinary bladder	Kidney	Lymphoma/multiple myeloma	Leukaemia	All sites
Males												
Africa	7.9	6.3	6.3	12.3	1.4	3.4	6.1	6.4	1.3	10.0	2.2	100
China	4.7	10.9	21.6	11.9	3.2	1.4	14.1	3.1	1.1	3.5	3.8	100
Asia, other	17.2	5.9	7.8	6.2	1.2	5.7	14.5	3.1	1.2	5.3	3.7	100
Polynesia/Micronesia	7.5	2.2	6.7	6.4	0.3	2.5	24.0	2.5	1.1	3.6	8.1	100
Latin America	6.1	4.0	13.5	1.5	2.1	3.9	12.9	4.2	1.7	5.5	3.6	100
Northern America	3.9	1.4	2.6	0.8	2.6	2.1	21.3	6.8	2.9	5.4	2.8	100
Former USSR	7.2	4.0	19.5	2.3	3.0	4.2	28.7	3.6	1.9	2.7	2.9	100
Europe	4.3	2.1	8.2	2.2	2.9	3.2	22.1	6.6	2.9	4.3	2.6	100
Japan	1.9	3.8	31.6	9.7	3.9	1.4	15.2	2.9	1.8	3.0	2.1	100
Australia/New Zealand	5.0	1.6	4.5	0.7	2.5	1.7	18.2	5.6	2.6	5.4	3.1	100
Developing countries	9.4	7.7	14.2	8.5	2.2	3.4	13.2	3.6	1.3	5.1	3.5	100
Developed countries	4.4	2.3	10.3	2.5	2.9	2.8	22.2	5.9	2.7	4.3	2.7	100
Females												
Africa	4.5	2.3	4.6	4.7	1.0	0.5	1.6	2.0	1.2	5.2	1.6	100
China	3.8	7.4	12.0	5.7	3.6	0.7	7.5	1.6	1.1	2.7	3.1	100
Asia, other	9.7	3.9	4.2	2.5	0.8	1.0	3.4	0.8	0.7	3.0	2.6	100
Polynesia/Micronesia	3.5	0.6	4.1	2.1	1.5	0.3	8.0	0.6	1.2	2.7	5.6	100
Latin America	1.8	1.3	7.0	1.2	1.4	0.5	3.5	1.1	1.0	3.9	2.6	100
Northern America	1.8	0.5	1.7	0.5	2.6	0.4	10.6	2.5	1.9	5.0	2.4	100
Former USSR	2.4	2.6	16.1	2.1	3.0	0.3	6.4	1.0	1.7	2.5	3.0	100
Europe	1.3	0.7	5.9	1.5	2.7	0.3	5.1	2.1	2.0	3.8	2.3	100
Japan	1.2	1.1	23.6	4.5	3.7	0.2	7.3	1.4	1.1	2.8	2.0	100
Australia/New Zealand	2.1	1.1	2.8	0.3	2.5	0.2	6.4	2.2	1.9	5.0	2.6	100
Developing countries	5.7	4.5	7.5	3.7	1.9	0.7	4.6	1.3	0.9	3.3	2.6	100
Developed countries	1.6	1.0	7.5	1.5	2.8	0.3	7.1	2.0	1.9	3.9	2.4	100

Overall mortality

The numbers of deaths from broad causes around 1985 were estimated by Bulatao and Stevens (1989) for developing and developed countries. Cancer accounts for 7% of the 37.9 million annual deaths occurring in the developing world; infectious and parasitic diseases are still the major cause of deaths, accounting for 36%. Figure 1 shows the distribution of causes of death by age in developing and developed countries, for the two sexes. The areas of the figures are proportional to the number of deaths occurring in the given age group, and the proportions of those due to cancer are shown in black. In developing countries, the importance of non-neoplastic causes of death in childhood is striking; nevertheless, a substantial proportion of deaths in adults and young adults are ascribed to cancer: 10% in the age group 15–44 and 21% in the age group 45–64 for either sex.

Table 4 shows the numbers of deaths and age-standardized rates of mortality for the 11 sites chosen and for all cancers estimated for 1985 (Pisani *et al.*, 1993). The estimated annual number of deaths is 2.1 million men and 1.9 million women. The

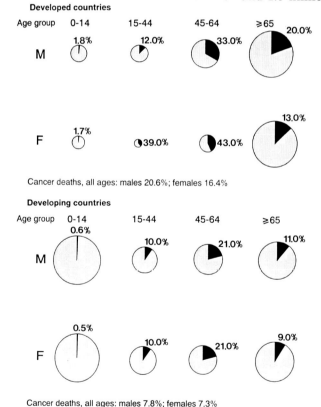

Figure 1. Distribution of deaths from cancer (black sectors) as percentage of all causes of death. Size of circle is proportional to the number of deaths in the relevant group.

Table 4. Numbers of deaths and age-standardized mortality rates per 100 000 person-years by site and region in 1985

Region	Oral cavity	Oesophagus	Stomach	Liver	Pancreas	Larynx	Lung	Urinary bladder	Kidney	Lymphoma/ multiple myeloma	Leukaemia	All sites
Male deaths												
Industrialized countries	34 678	40 607	147 211	44 485	52 900	27 598	365 959	39 287	26 867	44 057	39 179	1 224 653
Developing countries	71 058	85 152	137 124	85 815	22 865	19 611	135 989	25 050	8 025	28 295	21 713	840 768
Male age-standardized rates												
Industrialized countries	4.1	4.5	16.3	5.0	5.8	3.1	40.3	4.1	3.1	5.3	5.1	137.1
Developing countries	8.3	9.5	15.3	10.4	2.6	2.2	15.2	2.8	1.0	3.8	3.3	98.4
Female deaths												
Industrialized countries	10 610	15 509	108 048	28 843	49 894	2 746	104 327	14 525	18 872	38 169	33 875	1 000 331
Developing countries	58 365	66 223	98 244	50 173	29 863	6 424	63 648	13 273	7 566	25 468	19 433	902 481
Female age-standardized rates												
Industrialized countries	1.0	1.4	10.1	2.7	4.5	0.3	9.9	1.3	1.8	3.8	3.8	97.0
Developing countries	6.0	6.3	9.4	5.0	2.8	0.6	6.0	1.2	0.8	2.8	2.7	91.9

highly lethal cancers of the lung and stomach lead the list in men living in developed countries, giving age-standardized rates of 40.3 and 16.3; the corresponding figures for developing countries are 15.2 for lung and 13.3 for stomach cancer. In developing countries, the risk for cancer of the liver is also high, at 10.4.

Among women in both developed and developing countries, the most frequent cause of death from cancer among the sites studied is gastric cancer, with rates of 10.1 and 9.4, respectively. A similar risk (9.9) was estimated for lung cancer in industrialized countries. Death rates, like the incidence rates, from cancers of the oesophagus and mouth/pharynx in both men and women are remarkably high in developing countries.

Population aging and future burden of cancer

The burden of cancer is strongly affected by the age distribution of the population, and the age-standardized rates presented do not reflect the high proportion of young people living in developing regions. A dramatic growth of the populations in developing countries, accompanied by progressive aging of the population, is expected in the coming years (United Nations, 1991). The impact of such changes in the age distribution on the burden of cancer (assuming no change in standardized rates) is shown in Table 5. The number of cases is expected to double in developing countries by the year 2010, with relative increases of 98% in males and 97% in females. The epidemic is likely to be even more serious if no action is taken to prevent the spread of tobacco smoking in these areas.

Table 5. Numbers of incident cases, percentage increase and crude rates per 100 000 person-years expected in the years 2000 and 2010 on the basis of population growth and aging

Population	Year	No. of cases	Increase (%)	Crude rate
Males in developed countries	1985	1 872 000		329.6
	2000	2 344 000	25.2	380.1
	2010	2 720 000	45.3	424.0
Males in developing countries	1985	1 977 000		105.6
	2000	2 956 000	49.5	116.5
	2010	3 916 000	98.1	131.1
Females in developed countries	1985	1 787 000		294.8
	2000	2 087 000	16.8	322.4
	2010	2 316 000	29.6	346.7
Females in developing countries	1985	1 987 000		110.1
	2000	2 959 000	48.9	120.3
	2010	3 922 000	97.4	134.9

References

Bulatao, R.A. & Stevens, P.W. (1989) Estimates and projections of mortality by cause: a global overview, 1970–2015. In: Jamison, D.T. & Mosley, W.H., eds, *Evolving Health Sector Priorities in Developing Countries*, Washington DC, The World Bank, Population, Health and Nutrition Division

Devesa, S.S. & Fears, T. (1992) Non-Hodgkin's lymphoma time trends: United States and international data. *Cancer Res.*, **52**, 5432s–5440s

Parkin, D.M., Pisani, P. & Ferlay, J. (1993) Estimates of the worldwide incidence of 18 major cancers in 1985. *Int. J. Cancer*, **54**, 594–606

Pisani, P., Parkin, D.M. & Ferlay, J. (1993) Estimates of the worldwide mortality from 18 major cancers in 1985: implications for prevention and projections of future burden. *Int. J. Cancer*, **55**, 891–903

United Nations (1991) *World Population Prospects 1990* (Population Studies 120), New York, Department of International Economic and Social Affairs

Chapter 4. Identification of Occupational Carcinogens

H. Vainio, E. Matos and M. Kogevinas

Although current understanding of the relationship between occupational exposures and cancer is far from complete, increased risks have been associated with exposures in particular industries and occupations and to particular agents. Current knowledge on those occupational exposures that are considered to entail a carcinogenic risk to humans is summarized in the tables below. (Procedures for recognition and compensation of occupational cancer are not reviewed.)

Table 1 lists the industrial processes and occupations that have been evaluated with regard to their carcinogenic risk to humans in the *IARC Monographs*. The *Monographs* are an international source of information on chemicals, complex mixtures and industrial processes, providing detailed scientific reviews of available epidemiological and experimental data and evaluations of human carcinogenicity. The evaluation process results in a categorization of the carcinogenicity of agents (defined as including chemicals, groups of chemicals, complex mixtures and exposure circumstances) into one of five categories: (i) Group 1, the agent is carcinogenic to humans. (This category is normally used when there is sufficient evidence of carcinogenicity in humans.) (ii) Group 2A, the agent is probably carcinogenic to humans. (A positive association has been observed between the exposure and human cancer for which a causal interpretation is credible, but chance, bias or confounding could not be ruled out with reasonable confidence, and there is also sufficient evidence of carcinogenicity in experimental animals.) (iii) Group 2B, the agent is possibly carcinogenic to humans. (There is sufficient evidence of carcinogenicity in experimental animals but inadequate data on cancer in exposed humans.) (iv) Group 3, the agent, mixture or exposure circumstance is not classifiable as to its carcinogenicity to humans. (This grouping applies when no other category is used.) (v) Group 4, the agent, mixture or exposure circumstance is probably not carcinogenic to humans. (There is evidence suggesting lack of carcinogenicity in both humans and experimental animals.) The Table also indicates the probable target organs of the exposure.

Table 2 gives similar information with regard to chemicals, groups of chemicals and mixtures encountered predominantly in occupational settings; and Tables 3, 4 and 5 give pesticides, drugs and environmental agents to which there may be occupational exposure and that have been evaluated in the *IARC Monographs*. A number of occupations and industries for which there is evidence of an excess cancer risk have not yet been evaluated in the *IARC Monographs*. Tables 6 and 7 present more comprehensive lists of occupations and industries that have been associated in the scientific literature with an excess carcinogenic risk, with the relevant cancer sites and known or suspected causative agents. Table 6 presents industries and occupations in which the presence of a carcinogenic risk is considered to be well established, whereas Table 7 lists industrial processes and occupations in which an excess cancer risk has been reported but for which the evidence is not considered to be definitive. Table 7 includes some exposures already listed in Table 6 in relation to cancer sites for which there is inconclusive evidence of an association: For example, the asbestos production industry is included in Table 6 in relation to lung cancer and pleural and peritoneal mesothelioma and in Table 7 in relation to gastrointestinal neoplasms. The evidence in Tables 6 and 7 is based on the results of epidemiological studies of cancer risk in particular occupations; case reports, ecological studies and studies with no precise definition of occupation were not taken into account.

Table 1. Industrial processes and occupations associated with cancer in humans in *IARC Monographs* volumes 1–58

Group	Exposure	Target organ[a]
1	Aluminium production	Lung, bladder
	Auramine, manufacture of	Bladder
	Boot and shoe manufacture and repair	Nasal cavity, leukaemia
	Coal gasification	Skin, lung, bladder
	Coke production	Skin, lung, kidney
	Furniture and cabinet making	Nasal cavity
	Haematite mining (underground) with exposure to radon	Lung
	Iron and steel founding	Lung
	Isopropanol manufacture (strong-acid process)	Nasal cavity
	Magenta, manufacture of (1993)	Bladder
	Painter (occupational exposure as a) (1989)	Lung
	Rubber industry (certain occupations)	Bladder, leukaemia
	Strong-inorganic-acid mists containing sulfuric acid (occupational exposure to) (1992)	Lung, larynx
2A	Art glass, glass containers and pressed ware, manufacture of (1993)	(Lung, stomach)
	Hairdresser or barber (occupational exposure as a) (1993)	(Bladder, lung)
	Non-arsenical insecticides (occupational exposures in spraying and application of) (1991)	(Lung, myeloma)
	Petroleum refining (occupational exposures in) (1989)	(Leukaemia, skin)
2B	Carpentry and joinery	(Nasal cavity)
	Textile manufacturing industry (work in) (1990)	(Nasal cavity, bladder)

Evaluations confirmed or made in 1987 (IARC, 1987), except where noted by a date in parentheses.
[a] Suspected target organs are given in parentheses

Constructing (and interpreting) such lists of chemical and physical agents and associating them with specific occupations and industries is complicated by a number of factors: (i) Information on industrial processes and exposures is frequently poor and may not allow a complete evaluation of the importance of specific exposures.

Table 2. Chemicals, groups of chemicals and mixtures encountered predominantly in occupational settings that have been associated with cancer in humans in *IARC Monographs* volumes 1–58

Group	Exposure [Chemical Abstracts No.]	Target organ[a] Human	Animal[b]
1	4-Aminobiphenyl [92-67-1]	Bladder	M, Liver, bladder; R, Mammary gland, intestine; D/Rb, Bladder
	Arsenic [7440-38-2] and arsenic compounds[c]	Lung, skin	M/H, (Lung, larynx)
	Asbestos [1332-21-4]	Lung, pleura, peritoneum	M, Peritoneum (mesothelioma); R, Lung, pleura, peritoneum
	Benzene [71-43-2]	Leukaemia	M, Lung, lymphoma, leukaemia, Zymbal gland; R, Oral cavity, Zymbal gland, skin, mammary gland, forestomach
	Benzidine [92-87-5]	Bladder	M, Liver; R, Mammary gland, Zymbal gland; H, Liver
	Beryllium [7440-41-7] and beryllium compounds (1993)	Lung	R, Lung; Rb, Bone (osteosarcoma)
	Bis(chloromethyl)ether [542-88-1] and chloromethyl methyl ether [107-30-2] (technical-grade)	Lung	M, Lung, skin; R, Lung, nasal cavity; H, Lung
	Cadmium [7440-43-9] and cadmium compounds (1993)	Lung (prostate)	M, Testis (lung); R, Testis, lung, local, prostate
	Chromium[VI] compounds (1990)	Lung	M/R, Lung, local
	Coal-tar pitches [65996-93-2]	Skin, lung, bladder	M, Skin
	Coal-tars [8007-45-2]	Skin, lung	M/Rb, Skin; R, Lung
	Mineral oils, untreated and mildly-treated	Skin	M/Rb/Mk, Skin
	Mustard gas (Sulfur mustard) [505-60-2]	Pharynx, lung	M, (Lung, local)
	2-Naphthylamine [91-59-8]	Bladder	M, Lung, liver; R/H/D/Mk, Bladder
	Nickel compounds (1990)	Nasal cavity, lung	R, Lung, local
	Shale-oils [68308-34-9]	Skin (colon)	M/Rb, Skin
	Soots	Skin, lung	M, Skin; R, Lung
	Talc containing asbestiform fibres	Lung	—
	Vinyl chloride [75-01-4]	Liver, lung, blood vessels	M, Liver, lung, mammary gland, blood vessels; Zymbal gland, blood vessels; R, Liver, H, Liver, blood vessels, skin
2A	Acrylonitrile [107-13-1]	(Lung, prostate, lymphoma)	R, Zymbal gland, nervous system, mammary gland
	Benzidine-based dyes[d]	—	R, Liver, mammary gland, bladder
	1,3-Butadiene [106-99-0] (1992)	(Leukaemia, lymphoma)	M, Heart, lung, lymphoma, mammary gland, fore- stomach, ovary; R, Mammary gland, thyroid, pancreas

Table 2. (contd)

Group	Exposure [Chemical Abstracts No.]	Target organ[a] Human	Animal[b]
2A (contd)	para-Chloro-ortho-toluidine [95-69-2] and its strong-acid salts (1990)	(Bladder)	M, Blood vessels
	Creosotes [8001-58-9]	(Skin)	M, Skin, lung
	Diethyl sulfate[d] [64-67-5] (1992)	—	R, Forestomach, local, nervous system
	Dimethylcarbamoyl chloride[d] [79-44-7]	—	M, Skin, local; R/H, Nasal cavity
	Dimethyl sulfate[d] [77-78-1]	—	R, Nasal cavity, local, nervous system
	Epichlorohydrin[d] [106-89-8]	—	R, Forestomach, nasal cavity, lung
	Ethylene oxide[d] [75-21-8]	(Leukaemia)	M, Lung, local, mammary gland, lymphoma; R, Leukaemia, nervous system, peritoneum (mesothelioma) forestomach
	Formaldehyde [50-00-0]	(Nasopharynx)	R, Nasal cavity
	4,4'-Methylene bis(2-chloroaniline) (MOCA) [101-14-4] (1993)	(Bladder)	M, Liver; R, Liver, lung, mammary gland, Zymbal gland; D, Bladder
	Polychlorinated biphenyls [1336-36-3]	(Liver, bile ducts, leukaemia, lymphoma)	M/R, Liver
	Propylene oxide[d] [75-56-9]	—	M, Nasal cavity; R, Forestomach, nasal cavity
	Silica [14808-60-7], crystalline	(Lung)	R, Lung, lymphoma
	Styrene oxide[d] [96-09-3]	—	R, Forestomach
	Tris(2,3-dibromopropyl)phosphate[d] [126-72-7]	—	M, Forestomach, lung, liver, kidney
	Vinyl bromide[d] [593-60-2]	—	R, Liver, Zymbal gland
2B	Acetaldehyde [75-07-0]	—	R, Nasal cavity; H, Larynx
	Acetamide [60-35-5]	—	M, Lymphoma; R, Liver
	Acrylamide [79-06-1]	—	R, Mammary gland, adrenal, testis, thyroid
	para-Aminoazobenzene [60-09-3]	—	M, Liver, lymphoma, leukaemia; R, Liver, Skin
	ortho-Aminoazotoluene [97-56-3]	—	M, Liver, lung; R/H/Mk, Liver, bladder
	ortho-Anisidine [90-04-0]	—	M, Bladder, kidney; R, Kidney, thyroid
	Antimony trioxide [1309-64-4]	—	R, Lung
	Auramine [492-80-8] (technical-grade)	—	M/R, Liver
	Benzyl violet 4B [1694-09-3]	—	R, Skin, mammary gland
	Bitumens [8052-42-4], extracts of steam-refined and air-refined	—	M, Skin
	Bromodichloromethane [75-27-4] (1991)	—	M, Liver, kidney; R, Liver, kidney, colon
	β-Butyrolactone [3068-88-0]	—	M, Skin, local; R, Forestomach, local
	Carbon-black extracts	—	M, Skin

Table 2. (contd)

Group	Exposure [Chemical Abstracts No.]	Target organ[a]	
		Human	Animal[b]
2B (contd)	Carbon tetrachloride [56-23-5]	—	M/R, Liver
	Ceramic fibres (1988)	—	R, Pleura, peritoneum
	Chlorendic acid [115-28-6] (1990)	—	M, Liver, lung, thyroid; R, Liver, lung
	Chlorinated paraffins of average carbon chain length C$_{12}$ and average degree of chlorination approximately 60% (1990)	—	M, Liver, lung, thyroid; R, Liver, thyroid
	α-Chlorinated toluenes	—	M, Forestomach, skin, lung, oral cavity, oesophagus, stomach; R, Forestomach, thyroid
	para-Chloroaniline [106-47-8] (1993)	—	M, Blood vessels, liver; R, Spleen
	Chloroform [67-66-3]	—	M, Liver, kidney; R, Liver, kidney, thyroid
	4-Chloro-ortho-phenylenediamine [95-83-0]	—	M, Liver, R, Bladder
	CI Acid Red 114 [6459-94-5] (1993)	—	R, Skin, Zymbal gland, liver, clitoral gland, lung, oral cavity, intestine
	CI Basic Red 9 [569-61-9] (1993)	—	M, Liver, adrenal gland; R, Liver, local
	CI Direct Blue 15 [2429-74-5] (1993)	—	R, Skin, Zymbal gland, liver, intestine, oral cavity, leukaemia, preputial gland, uterus, uterus, clitoral gland
	Cobalt [7440-48-4] and cobalt compounds (1991)	—	R, Lung, local/peritoneum, pleura
	para-Cresidine [120-71-8]	—	M/R, Liver, bladder
	N,N'-Diacetylbenzidine [613-35-4]	—	R, Liver, Zymbal gland, mammary gland
	2,4-Diaminoanisole [615-05-4]	—	M, Thyroid; R, Skin, clitoral gland, preputial gland, Zymbal gland, thyroid
	4,4'-Diaminodiphenyl ether [101-80-4]	—	M/R, Liver, thyroid
	2,4-Diaminotoluene [95-80-7]	—	M, Liver, lymphoma; R, Liver, mammary gland
	para-Dichlorobenzene [106-46-7]	—	M, Liver, R, Kidney
	3,3'-Dichlorobenzidine [91-94-1]	—	M, Liver, leukaemia; R, Mammary gland, Zymbal gland, leukaemia; H/D, Bladder
	3,3'-Dichloro-4,4'-diaminodiphenyl ether [28434-86-8]	—	R, Zymbal gland
	1,2-Dichloroethane [107-06-2]	—	M, Lung, lymphoma, liver, mammary gland, uterus; R, Forestomach, mammary gland, blood vessels
	Dichloromethane [75-09-2]	—	M, Lung, liver; R, Mammary gland
	Diepoxybutane [1464-53-5]	—	M, Skin, lung, local

Table 2. (contd)

Group	Exposure [Chemical Abstracts No.]	Target organ[a] Human	Animal[b]
2B (contd)	Diesel fuel, marine (1989)	—	M, Skin
	Di(2-ethylhexyl)phthalate [117-81-7]	—	M/R, Liver
	1,2-Diethylhydrazine [1615-80-1]	—	R, Liver, mammary gland, brain
	Diglycidyl resorcinol ether [101-90-6]	—	M, Forestomach, liver; R, Forestomach
	Diisopropyl sulfate [2973-10-6] (1992)	—	M, Skin; R, Local
	3,3′-Dimethoxybenzidine (*ortho*-Dianis·dine) [119-90-4]	—	R, Zymbal gland, bladder, intestine, skin
	para-Dimethylaminoazobenzene [60-11-7] (1993)	—	M, Liver, local; R, Liver, skin; D, Bladder
	2,6-Dimethylaniline (2,6-Xylidine) [87-62-7] (1993)	—	R, Nasal cavity, skin, liver
	3,3′-Dimethylbenzidine (*ortho*-Tolidine) [119-93-7]	—	R, Zymbal gland, mammary gland
	Dimethylformamide [68-12-2] (1989)	(Testis)	—
	1,1-Dimethylhydrazine [57-14-7]	—	M, Lung, liver, kidney, blood vessels
	1,2-Dimethylhydrazine [540-73-8]	—	M, Lung, liver, blood vessels, intestine; R, Intestine, liver; H, Intestine, liver, blood vessels
	1,4-Dioxane [123-91-1]	—	R, Liver, nasal cavity; G, Liver/bile duct
	Disperse Blue 1 [2475-45-8] (1990)	—	M, Lung; R, Bladder
	Ethyl acrylate [140-88-5]	—	M/R, Forestomach
	Ethylene thiourea [96-45-7]	—	M, Liver; R, Thyroid
	Fuel oils, residual (heavy) (1989)	—	M, Skin
	Gasoline[e] (1989)	—	M, Liver; R, (Kidney)
	Glasswool (1988)	—	R, Lung, pleura, peritoneum; H, Pleura
	Glycidaldehyde [765-34-4]	—	M, Skin, local; R, Local
	HC Blue No. 1 [2784-94-3] (1993)	—	M, Liver (thyroid); R, Lung
	Hexamethylphosphoramide [680-31-9]	—	R, Nasal cavity
	Hydrazine [302-01-2]	—	M, Lung, liver, lymphoma/leukaemia; R, Liver, lung, nasal cavity
	Lead [7439-92-1] and lead compounds, inorganic	—	M, Kidney; R, Kidney, brain
	2-Methylaziridine [75-55-8]	—	R, Mammary gland, leukaemia, intestine, Zymbal gland
	4,4′-Methylene bis(2-methylaniline) [838-88-0]	—	R, Liver, lung, skin, mammary gland; D, Liver, lung
	4,4′-Methylenedianiline [101-77-9]	—	M/R, Liver, thyroid
	Methylmercury compounds (1993)	—	M, Kidney
	2-Methyl-1-nitroanthraquinone [129-15-7] (uncertain purity)	—	M, Blood vessels; R, Liver, blood vessels, subcutis

Table 2. (contd)

Group	Exposure [Chemical Abstracts No.]	Target organ[a] Human	Animal[b]
2B (contd)	Nickel, metallic [7440-02-0] (1990)	—	R, Lung, pleura, local
	Nitrilotriacetic acid [139-13-9] and its salts (1990)	—	R, Kidney, bladder
	5-Nitroacenaphthene [602-87-9]	—	R, Mammary gland, intestine; H, Bile duct
	2-Nitropropane [79-46-9]	—	R, Liver
	N-Nitrosodiethanolamine [1116-54-7]	—	R, Liver, kidney; H, Lung, nasal cavity, liver
	Oil Orange SS [2646-17-5]	—	M, Intestine, bladder
	Phenylglycidyl ether [122-60-1] (1989)	—	R, Nasal cavity
	Polybrominated biphenyls [Firemaster BP-6, 59536-65-1]	—	M/R, Liver
	Ponceau MX [3761-53-3]	—	M, Liver, intestine; R, Liver
	Ponceau 3R [3564-09-8]	—	M, Bladder; R, Liver
	1,3-Propane sultone [1120-71-4]	—	R, Brain, local
	β-Propiolactone [57-57-8]	—	M, Skin, local; R, Forestomach
	Rockwool (1988)	(Lung)	R, Pleura, peritoneum
	Slagwool (1988)	(Lung)	—
	Styrene[e] [100-42-5]	—	M, (Lung)
	2,3,7,8-Tetrachlorodibenzo-para-dioxin (TCDD) [1746-01-6]	—	M, Liver, thyroid; R, Liver, lung, nasal cavity, tongue, thyroid
	Tetrachloroethylene [127-18-4]	—	M, Liver; R, Leukaemia
	Thioacetamide [62-55-5]	—	M/R, Liver
	4,4'-Thiodianiline [139-65-1]	—	M, Liver, thyroid; R, Liver, Zymbal gland, uterus, thyroid
	Thiourea [62-56-6]	—	R, Liver, thyroid, Zymbal gland
	Toluene diisocyanates [26471-62-5]	—	M, Blood vessels; R, Subcutis, spleen, bladder, mammary gland
	ortho-Toluidine [95-53-4]	—	R, Liver, lymphoma, local
	Trypan blue [72-57-1]	—	R, Liver, local
	Welding fumes (1990)	(Lung)	—

Evaluations confirmed or made in 1987 (IARC, 1987), except where noted by a date in parentheses

a Suspected target organs are given in parentheses.
b M, mouse; R, rat; H, hamster; Mk, monkey; G, guinea-pig; D, dog; Rb, rabbit
c This evaluation applies to the group of chemicals as a whole and not necessarily to all individual chemicals within the group.
d Overall evaluation changed from 2B to 2A with supporting evidence from other relevant data
e Overall evaluation changed from 3 to 2B with supporting evidence from other relevant data

Table 3. Pesticides that have been associated with cancer in humans in *IARC Monographs volumes 1–58*

Group	Exposure [Chemical Abstracts No.]	Target organ[a] Human	Animal[b]
2A	Captafol[c] [2425-06-1] (1991)	—	M, Heart, intestine, liver, kidney; R, Liver, kidney
	Ethylene dibromide[c] [106-93-4]	—	M, Forestomach, lung, skin; R, Forestomach, liver, blood vessels, nasal cavity, peritoneum, mammary gland, skin
2B	Amitrole [61-82-5]	—	M/R, Liver, thyroid
	Aramite® [140-57-8]	—	M/R/D, Liver/bile duct
	Atrazine[d] [1912-24-9] (1991)	—	R, Mammary gland, uterus, leukaemia/lymphoma
	Chlordane [57-74-9] (1991)	—	M, Liver; R, Liver, thyroid
	Chlordecone (Kepone) [143-50-0]	—	M/R, Liver
	Chlorophenols	(Soft-tissue sarcoma)	M, Liver; R, Lymphoma/leukaemia
	Chlorophenoxy herbicides	(Sarcoma, lymphoma)	–
	DDT [50-29-3] (1991)	—	M, Liver, lymphoma; R, Liver; H, Adrenal
	1,2-Dibromo-3-chloropropane [96-12-8]	—	M, Forestomach, nasal cavity, lung; R, Forestomach, mammary gland, nasal cavity
	1,3-Dichloropropene (technical-grade) [542-75-6]	—	M, Lung, forestomach, bladder; R, Forestomach, liver
	Dichlorvos [62-73-7] (1991)	—	M, Forestomach, oesophagus; R, Forestomach, pancreas, leukaemia
	Heptachlor [76-44-8] (1991)	—	M, Liver; R, Thyroid
	Hexachlorobenzene [118-74-1]	—	M/R/H, Liver
	Hexachlorocyclohexanes (HCH)	—	M, Liver, lymphoma; R, Liver, thyroid
	Mirex [2385-85-5]	—	M/R, Liver
	Nitrofen [1836-75-5] (technical-grade)	—	M, Liver, blood vessels; R, Pancreas
	Pentachlorophenol [87-86-5] (1991)	—	M, Liver
	Sodium *ortho*-phenylphenate [132-27-4]	—	M, Liver; R, Bladder
	Sulfallate [95-06-7]	—	M, Lung, mammary gland; R, Forestomach, mammary gland
	Toxaphene (Polychlorinated camphenes) [8001-35-2] (1979)	—	M, Liver; R, Thyroid

Evaluations confirmed or made in 1987 (IARC, 1987), except where noted by a date in parentheses.

[a] Suspected target organs are given in parentheses.

[b] M, mouse; R, rat; H, hamster; Mk, monkey; G, guinea-pig; D, dog; Rb, rabbit

[c] Overall evaluation changed from 2B to 2A with supporting evidence from other relevant data

[d] Overall evaluation changed from 3 to 2B with supporting evidence from other relevant data

Table 4. Drugs that have been associated with cancer in humans in *IARC Monographs* volumes 1–58

Group	Exposure [Chemical Abstracts No.]	Target organ[a] Human	Animal[b]
1	Analgesic mixtures containing phenacetin	Kidney, bladder	R, Kidney
	Azathioprine [446-86-6]	Lymphoma, hepatobiliary system, skin	M, (Lymphoma); R (Zymbal gland)
	N,N-Bis(2-chloroethyl)-2-naphthylamine (Chlornaphazine) [494-03-1]	Bladder	M, (Lung); R, (Local)
	1,4-Butanediol dimethanesulfonate (Myleran) [55-98-1]	Leukaemia	M, Lymphoma/leukaemia, ovary
	Chlorambucil [305-03-3]	Leukaemia	M, (Lung); R, Lymphoma/leukaemia
	1-(2-Chloroethyl)-3-(4-methylcyclohexyl)-1-nitrosourea (Methyl-CCNU) [13909-09-6]	Leukaemia	R, (Lung)
	Ciclosporin [79217-60-0] (1990)	Lymphoma, skin	M, (Leukaemia)
	Cyclophosphamide [50-18-0] [6055-19-2]	Leukaemia, bladder	M, Leukaemia, lung, mammary gland; R, Bladder, leukaemia
	Diethylstilboestrol [56-53-1]	Cervix/vagina, breast	M, Mammary gland, cervix, uterus, ovary, lymphoma; R, Mammary gland, pituitary; H, Kidney, cervix, uterus
	Melphalan [148-82-3]	Leukaemia	M, Lymphoma, lung
	8-Methoxypsoralen (Methoxsalen) [298-81-7] plus ultraviolet radiation	Skin	M, Skin
	MOPP and other combined chemotherapy including alkylating agents	Leukaemia	—
	Oestrogen replacement therapy	Uterus	—
	Oestrogens, nonsteroidal[c]	Cervix/vagina, breast	—
	Oestrogens, steroidal[c]	Uterus	—
	Oral contraceptives, combined[d]	Liver	—
	Oral contraceptives, sequential	Uterus	—
	Thiotepa [52-24-4] (1990)	Leukaemia	M/R, Leukaemia
	Treosulfan [299-75-2]	Leukaemia	—

Table 4. (contd)

Group	Exposure [Chemical Abstracts No.]	Target organ[a]	
		Human	Animal[b]
2A	Adriamycin[e] [23214-92-8]	—	R, Mammary gland
	Androgenic (anabolic) steroids	(Liver)	R, Prostate
	Azacitidine[e] [320-67-2] (1990)	—	M, Lung, lymphoma, leukaemia
	Bischloroethyl nitrosourea (BCNU) [154-93-8]	(Leukaemia)	R, Lung, nervous system
	Chloramphenicol[e] [56-75-7] (1990)	(Leukaemia)	—
	1-(2-Chloroethyl)-3-cyclohexyl-1-nitrosourea (CCNU) [13010-47-4]	—	R, Lung
	Chlorozotocin[e] [54749-90-5] (1990)	—	R, Peritoneum
	Cisplatin[e] [15663-27-1] (1987)	—	M, Lung; R, Leukaemia
	5-Methoxypsoralen[e] [484-20-8]	—	M, Skin
	Nitrogen mustard [51-75-2]	(Skin)	M, Lung, skin
	Phenacetin [62-44-2]	(Kidney, bladder)	M, Kidney; R, Kidney, bladder, nasal cavity
	Procarbazine hydrochloride[e] [366-70-1]	—	M, Lung, leukaemia; R, Mammary gland, brain, leukaemia; Mk, leukaemia
2B	2-Amino-5-(5-nitro-2-furyl)-1,3,4-thiadiazole [712-68-5]	—	R, Mammary gland
	Azaserine [115-02-6]	—	R, Pancreas, kidney
	Bleomycins[f] [11056-06-7]	—	R (Kidney)
	Dacarbazine [4342-03-4]	—	M, Lung, uterus, lymphoma; R, Mammary gland, lymphoma, brain
	Dantron (Chrysazin; 1,8-Dihydroxyanthraquinone) [117-10-2] (1990)	—	M, Liver, intestine
	Daunomycin [20830-81-3]	—	R, Mammary gland, kidney
	trans-2-[(Dimethylamino)methylimino]-5-[2-(5-nitro-2-furyl)vinyl]-1,3,4-oxadiazole [25962-77-0]	—	R, Forestomach, mammary gland
	Griseofulvin [126-07-8]	—	M, Liver, local
	Iron–dextran complex [9004-66-4]	—	R, Local
	Medroxyprogesterone acetate [71-58-9]	—	M, Liver, mammary gland, cervix; R, Pituitary, ovary, mammary gland, liver; D, Mammary gland
	Merphalan [531-76-0]	—	R, Mammary gland

Table 4 (contd)

Group	Exposure [Chemical Abstracts No.]	Target organ[a]	
		Human	Animal[b]
2B (contd)	Methylthiouracil [56-04-2]	—	M/R, Thyroid
	Metronidazole [443-48-1]	—	M, Lung, lymphoma; R, Mammary gland, pituitary, testis, liver
	Mitomycin C [50-07-7]	—	M, Local; R, Mammary gland, lung, local
	5-(Morpholinomethyl)-3-[(5-nitrofurfurylidene)-amino]-2-oxazolidinone [3795-88-8]	—	R, Mammary gland, lymphoma
	Nafenopin [3771-19-5]	—	M/R, Liver
	Niridazole [61-57-4]	—	M, Lung, forestomach, mammary gland, bladder; H, Forestomach, bladder
	1-[(5-Nitrofurfurylidene)amino]-2-imidazolidinone [555-84-0]	—	R, Mammary gland, lymphoma
	N-[4-(5-Nitro-2-furyl)-2-thiazolyl]acetamide [531-82-8]	—	M, Forestomach, leukaemia; R, Mammary gland, kidney, lung; H, Forestomach, bladder
	Panfuran S (containing dihydroxymethylfuratrizine [794-93-4])	—	M/R, Forestomach, intestine
	Phenazopyridine hydrochloride [136-40-3]	—	M, Liver; R, Colon/rectum
	Phenobarbital [50-06-6]	—	M/R, Liver
	Phenoxybenzamine hydrochloride [63-92-3]	—	M, Lung, peritoneum; R, Peritoneum
	Phenytoin [57-41-0]	(Brain, lymphoma)	M, (Lymphoma)
	Trichlormethine (Trimustine hydrochloride) [817-09-4] (1990)	—	R, Local, intestine
	Uracil mustard [66-75-1]	—	M, Lung, liver, ovary, lymphoma; R, Lymphoma, pancreas, ovary, mammary gland
	Urethane [51-79-6]	—	M, Lung, liver, skin, mammary gland; R, Liver, blood vessels; H, Skin, forestomach, blood vessels, mammary gland

Evaluations confirmed or made in 1987 (IARC, 1987), except where noted by a date in parentheses

[a] Suspected target organs are given in parentheses.

[b] i., mouse; R, rat; H, hamster; Mk, monkey; D, dog

[c] This evaluation applies to the group of chemicals as a whole and not necessarily to all individual chemicals within the group.

[d] There is also conclusive evidence that these agents have a protective effect against cancers of the ovary and endometrium.

[e] Overall evaluation changed from 2B to 2A with supporting evidence from other relevant data

[f] Overall evaluation changed from 3 to 2B with supporting evidence from other relevant data

Table 5. Environmental agents and exposures which may be encountered in occupational settings and have been associated with cancer in humans in *IARC Monographs* volumes 1–58

Group	Exposure [Chemical Abstracts No.]	Target organ[a]	
		Human	Animal[b]
1	Aflatoxins [1402-68-2] (1993)	Liver	M, Lung, liver; R, Liver, local, kidney, colon; Mk, Liver, bone, gall-bladder, pancreas; H/F/Dk, Liver
	Erionite [66733-21-9]	Pleura	M, Local; R, Pleura, local
	Radon [10043-92-2] and its decay products (1988)	Lung	R/D, Lung
	Solar radiation (1992)	Skin	M, Skin
	Tobacco smoke	Lung, bladder, oral cavity, pharynx, larynx, oesophagus, pancreas	R/H, Lung; M/Rb, Skin
2A	Benz[a]anthracene[c] [56-55-3]	—	M, Lung, liver, skin, bladder
	Benzo[a]pyrene[c] [50-32-8]	—	M, Forestomach, lung, skin; R, Forestomach, mammary gland; H, Forestomach; Rb, Skin
	Dibenz[a,h]anthracene[c] [52-70-3]	—	M, Forestomach, lung, skin, mammary gland
	Diesel engine exhaust (1989)	(Lung, bladder)	M, Lung, skin; R, Lung
	IQ[c] (2-Amino-3-methylimidazo[4,5-f]quinoline) [76180-96-6] (1993)	—	M, Liver, lung, forestomach; R, Liver, intestine, Zymbal gland, mammary gland, clitoral gland, skin; Mk, Liver
	N-Nitrosodimethylamine[c] [62-75-9]	—	M, Liver, lung, kidney, blood vessels; R, Liver/bile duct, blood vessels, kidney, lung, nasal cavity; H, Bile duct, blood vessels; G, Liver/bile duct; F, Liver
	Ultraviolet radiation A[c] (1992)	(Skin)	M, Skin
	Ultraviolet radiation B[c] (1992)	(Skin)	M, Skin
	Ultraviolet radiation C[c] (1992)	(Skin)	M, Skin

Table 5. (contd)

Group	Exposure [Chemical Abstracts No.]	Target organ[a]	
		Human	Animal[b]
2B	Aflatoxin M$_1$ [6795-23-9] (1993)	—	R/F, Liver
	Benzo[b]fluoranthene [205-99-2]	—	M, Skin, local
	Benzo[j]fluoranthene [205-82-3]	—	M, Skin; R, Lung
	Benzo[k]fluoranthene [207-08-9]	—	M, Skin; R, Lung
	Dibenz[a,h]acridine [226-36-8]	—	M, Skin, lung
	Dibenz[a,j]acridine [224-42-0]	—	M, Sking, lung
	Dibenzo[a,e]pyrene [192-65-4]	—	M, Skin
	Dibenzo[a,h]pyrene [189-64-0]	—	M, Skin, local
	Dibenzo[a,i]pyrene [189-55-9]	—	M, Skin, local
	Dibenzo[a,l]pyrene [191-30-0]	—	M, Skin, local
	1,6-Dinitropyrene [42397-64-8] (1989)	—	M, Liver, lung; R, Lung, local, leukaemia; G, Lung
	1,8-Dinitropyrene [42397-65-9] (1989)	—	M, Liver; R, Mammary gland, leukaemia
	Engine exhaust, gasoline (1989)	—	M, Skin; R, Lung
	5-Methylchrysene [3697-24-3]	—	M, Skin, local
	2-Nitrofluorene [607-57-8] (1989)	—	R, Mammary gland, liver, leukaemia, forestomach
	1-Nitropyrene [5522-43-0] (1989)	—	M, Lung, liver; R, Mammary gland
	4-Nitropyrene [57835-92-4] (1989)	—	M, Liver, lung; R, Mammary gland
	N-Nitrosomorpholine [59-89-2]	—	M, Liver, blood vessels; R, Liver/bile duct, kidney, blood vessels; H, Trachea, nasal cavity, oesophagus
	Ochratoxin A [303-47-9] (1993)	(Urothelial urinary tract)	M, Liver, kidney; R, Kidney
	Toxins derived from *Fusarium moniliforme* (1993)	(Oesophagus)	R, Liver, forestomach, oesophagus

Evaluations confirmed or made in 1987 (IARC, 1987), except where noted by a date in parentheses

[a] Suspected target organs are given in parentheses.

[b] M, mouse; R, rat; H, hamster; Mk, monkey; G, guinea-pig; D, dog; Rb, rabbit; F, fish; Dk, duck

[c] Overall evaluation changed from 2B to 2A with supporting evidence from other relevant data

Table 6. Occupations and industries recognized as presenting a carcinogenic risk

Industry (ISIC code)	Occupation/process	Cancer site/type	Known (or suspected) causative agent
Agriculture, forestry and fishing (1)	Vineyard workers using arsenical insecticides	Lung, skin	Arsenic compounds
	Fishermen	Skin, lip	Ultraviolet radiation
Mining and quarrying (2)	Arsenic mining	Lung, skin	Arsenic compounds
	Iron-ore (haematite) mining	Lung	Radon decay products
	Asbestos mining	Lung, pleural and peritoneal mesothelioma	Asbestos
	Uranium mining	Lung	Radon decay products
	Talc mining and milling	Lung	Talc containing asbestiform fibres
Chemical (35)	Bis(chloromethyl) ether (BCME) and chloro-methyl methyl ether (CMME) production workers and users	Lung (oat-cell carcinoma)	BCME, CMME
	Vinyl chloride production	Liver angiosarcoma	Vinyl chloride monomer
	Isopropyl alcohol manufacture (strong-acid process)	Sinonasal	Not identified
	Pigment chromate production	Lung, sinonasal	Chromium[VI] compounds
	Dye manufacture and use	Bladder	Benzidine, 2-naphthylamine, 4-aminobiphenyl
	Auramine manufacture	Bladder	Auramine and other aromatic amines used in the process)
	para-Chloro-ortho-toluidine production	Bladder	para-Chloro-ortho-toluidine and its strong-acid salts
Leather (324)	Boot and shoe manufacture	Sinonasal, leukaemia	Leather dust, benzene
Wood and wood products (33)	Furniture and cabinet makers	Sinonasal	Wood dust
Pesticides and herbicides production (3512)	Arsenical insecticides production and packaging	Lung	Arsenic compounds
Rubber (355)	Rubber manufacture	Leukaemia	Benzene
		Bladder	Aromatic amines
	Calendering, tyre curing, tyre building	Leukaemia	Benzene

Table 6. (contd)

Industry (ISIC code)	Occupation/process	Cancer site/type	Known (or suspected) causative agent
Rubber (contd)	Millers, mixers	Bladder	Aromatic amines
	Synthetic latex production, tyre curing, calender operatives, reclaim, cable makers	Bladder	Aromatic amines
	Rubber film production	Leukaemia	Benzene
Asbestos production (3699)	Insulated material production (pipes, sheeting, textile clothes, masks, asbestos—cement products)	Lung, pleural and peritoneal mesothelioma	Asbestos
Metals (37)	Aluminium production	Lung, bladder	Polycyclic aromatic hydrocarbons, tar volatiles
	Copper smelting	Lung	Arsenic compounds
	Chromate production	Lung, sinonasal	Chromium[VI] compounds
	Chromium plating	Lung, sinonasal	Chromium[VI] compounds
	Iron and steel founding	Lung	Not identified
	Nickel refining	Sinonasal, lung	Nickel compounds
	Pickling operations	Larynx, lung	Inorganic acid mists containing sulfuric acid
	Cadmium production and refining; nickel-cadmium battery manufacture; cadmium pigment manufacture; cadmium alloy production; electroplating; zinc smelters; brazing and polyvinyl chloride compounding	Lung	Cadmium and cadmium compounds
	Beryllium refining and machining; production of beryllium-containing products	Lung	Beryllium and beryllium compounds
Shipbuilding, motor vehicle and railroad equipment manufacture (385)	Shipyard and dockyard, motor vehicle and railroad manufacture workers	Lung, pleural and peritoneal mesothelioma	Asbestos
Gas (4)	Coke plant workers	Lung	Benzo[a]pyrene
	Gas workers	Lung, bladder, scrotum	Coal carbonization products, β-naphthylamine
	Gas-retort house workers	Bladder	β-Naphthylamine
Construction (5)	Insulators and pipe coverers	Lung, pleural and peritoneal mesothelioma	Asbestos
	Roofers, asphalt workers	Lung	Polycyclic aromatic hydrocarons
Other	Medical personnel	Skin, leukaemia	Ionizing radiation
	Painters (construction, automotive industry and other users)	Lung	Not identified

Table 7. Occupations and industries reported to present a cancer excess but for which the assessment of the carcinogenic risk is not definitive

Industry (ISIC code)	Occupation/process	Cancer site/type	Known (or suspected) causative agent
Agriculture, forestry and fishing (1)	Farmers, farm workers	Lymphatic and haematopoietic system (leukaemia, lymphoma)	Not identified
	Herbicide application	Malignant lymphomas, soft-tissue sarcomas	Chlorophenoxy herbicides, chlorophenols (presumably contaminated with poly-chlorinated dibenzodioxins)
	Insecticide application	Lung, lymphoma	Non-arsenical insecticides
Mining and quarrying (2)	Zinc–lead mining	Lung	Radon decay products
	Coal	Stomach	Coal dust
	Metal mining	Lung	Crystalline silica
	Asbestos mining	Gastrointestinal tract	Asbestos
Textile manufacture (321)	Dyers	Bladder	Dyes
	Weavers	Bladder, sinonasal	Dusts from fibres and yarns
Leather (323)	Tanners and processors	Bladder, pancreas, lung	Leather dust, other chemicals, chromium
	Boot and shoe manufacture and repair	Sinonasal, stomach, bladder	Not identified
Wood, wood products (33), pulp and paper (341)	Lumbermen and sawmill workers	Nasal cavity, Hodgkin's lymphoma	Wood dust, chlorophenols
	Pulp and papermill workers	Lymphopoietic tissue, lung	Not identified
	Carpenters, joiners	Nasal cavity, Hodgkin's lymphoma	Wood dust, solvents
	Woodworkers unspecified	Lymphomas	Not identified
	Plywood production/particle-board production	Nasopharynx, sinonasal	Formaldehyde
Printing (342)	Rotogravure workers, binders, printing press-men, machine-room workers and other jobs	Lymphocytic and haematopoietic system, buccal cavity, lung, kidney	Oil mist, solvents
Chemical (35)	1,3-Butadiene production	Lymphatic and haematopoietic system	1,3-Butadiene
	Acrylonitrile production	Lung, colon	Acrylonitrile

Table 7. (contd)

Industry (ISIC code)	Occupation/process	Cancer site/type	Known (or suspected) causative agent
Chemical (contd)	Vinylidene chloride production	Lung	Vinylidene chloride (mixed exposure with acrylonitrile)
	Isopropyl alcohol manufacture (strong-acid process)	Larynx	Not identified
	Polychloroprene production	Lung	Chloroprene
	Dimethylsulfate production	Lung	Dimethylsulfate
	Epichlorohydrin production	Lung, lymphatic and haematopoietic system (leukaemia)	Epichlorohydrin
	Ethylene oxide production	Lymphatic and haematopoietic system (leukaemia), stomach	Ethylene oxide
	Ethylene dibromide production	Digestive system	Ethylene dibromide
	Formaldehyde production	Nasopharynx, sinonasal	Formaldehyde
	Flame retardant and plasticizer use	Skin (melanoma)	Polychlorinated biphenyls
	Benzoyl chloride production	Lung	Benzoyl chloride
Herbicides production (3512)	Chlorophenoxy herbicide production	Soft-tissue sarcoma	Chlorophenoxy herbicides, chlorophenols (contaminated with polychlorinated dibenzo-dioxins)
Petroleum (353)	Petroleum refining	Skin, leukaemia, brain	Benzene, polycyclic [?aromatic] hydrocarbons, untreated and mildly treated mineral oils
Rubber (355)	Various occupations in rubber manufacture	Lymphoma, multiple myeloma, stomach, brain, lung	Not identified
	Styrene–butadiene rubber production	Lymphatic and haematopoietic system	1,3-Butadiene
Ceramic, glass and refractory brick (36)	Ceramic and pottery workers	Lung	Crystalline silica
	Glass workers (art glass, container and pressed ware)	Lung	Arsenic and other metal oxides, silica, polycyclic aromatic hydrocarbons

Table 7. (contd)

Industry (ISIC code)	Occupation/process	Cancer site/type	Known (or suspected) causative agent
Asbestos production (3699)	Insulation material production (pipes, sheeting, textiles, clothes, masks, asbestos cement products)	Larynx, gastrointestinal tract	Asbestos
Metals (37, 38)	Smelting	Respiratory and digestive system	Lead compounds
	Cadmium production and refining; nickel–cadmium battery manufacture; cadmium pigment manufacture; cadmium alloy production; electroplating; zinc, smelting; brazing and polyvinyl chloride compounding	Prostate	Cadmium and cadmium compounds
	Iron and steel founding	Lung	Crystalline silica
Shipbuilding (384)	Shipyard and dockyard workers	Larynx, digestive system	Asbestos
Transport (7)	Railroad workers, filling station attendants, bus and truck drivers, operators of excavating machines	Lung, bladder	Diesel engine exhaust
Construction (5)	Insulators and pipe coverers	Larynx, gastrointestinal tract	Asbestos
	Roofers, asphalt workers	Mouth, pharynx, larynx, oesophagus, stomach	Benzo[a]pyrene, other pitch volatile agents
Professionals	Embalmers, medical personnel	Sinonasal, nasopharynx	Formaldehyde
Other	Radium dial workers	Breast	Radon
	Laundry and dry cleaners using carbon tetrachloride	Lung, skin, cervix uteri	Tri- and tetrachloroethylene

(ii)Exposures to well-known carcinogenic agents, such as vinyl chloride and benzene, occur at different intensities in different occupational situations. (iii) Exposures in a given occupational situation change over time, either because identified carcinogenic agents are substituted by other agents or (more frequently) because new industrial processes or materials are introduced. (iv) Any such list can refer only to the relatively small number of exposures that have been investigated with respect to the presence of a carcinogenic risk. (v) Most studies of carcinogenic exposures in the occupational environment have been conducted in industrially developed countries, where exposures were relatively high in the past but are now generally lower than those encountered in industries in developing countries. The most critical limitation of a classification of this type, however, and in particular its generalization to all areas of the world, is that the presence of a carcinogen in an occupational situation does not necessarily mean that workers are exposed to it, and, in contrast, the absence of identified carcinogens does not exclude the presence of yet unidentified causes of cancer.

A particular problem in developing countries is that much industrial activity takes place in small occupational settings (see Chapter 6), which are often characterized by old machinery, unsafe buildings, employees with limited training and education and employers with limited financial resources. Protective clothing, respirators, gloves and other safety equipment are seldom available or used. Such small companies tend to be scattered geographically and inaccessible to inspectors from health and safety enforcement agencies. The widespread development of industry therefore means that the prevalence of significant occupational exposures has probably never been greater than it is today. For instance, one-third of the adult urban Chinese population reported a history of occupational exposure to dust, and one million Chinese have pneumoconiosis due to exposure to silica (LaDou, 1991).

Virtually all of the occupations and industries listed in Tables 6 and 7 have been studied formally, in terms of cancer risk, only in the developed world. Most of them, however, also exist in developing countries, where exposure levels may be higher: The processes used are often more polluting and of types no longer used in industrialized nations; evidence from some epidemiological studies may in fact relate primarily to the higher levels of exposure that occurred in developed countries in the past. An important factor in developing countries is the low level of awareness, both among workers and management, about the carcinogenic hazards of occupational exposures, as such information is generally poorly disseminated and managed. Furthermore, as noted above, occupational carcinogens may have greater effects on people with poor living conditions and poor diets than on healthy people.

References

IARC (1987) *IARC Monographs on the Evaluation of Carcinogenic Risks to Humans*, Suppl. 7, *Overall Evaluations of Carcinogenicity to Humans: An Updating of* IARC Monographs *Volumes 1 to 42*, Lyon
LaDou, J. (1991) The export of industrial hazards to developing countries. In: Jeyaratnam, J., ed., *Occupational Health in Developing Countries*, Oxford, Oxford University Press, pp. 340–358

Part II

Exposure

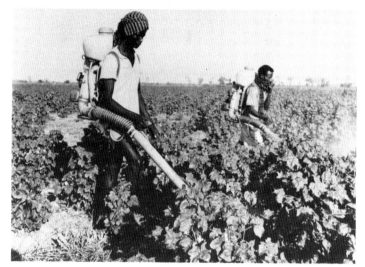

African farmers spraying insecticides without protective masks or clothing.
Photo: Courtesy of World Health Organization and Food and Agriculture Organization

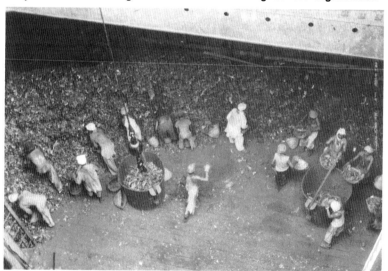

Unloading metal waste from the hold of a freighter in Pakistan leads to heavy exposure to metallic dusts

Photos: Courtesy of International Labour Office

Chapter 5. Occupational Exposure to Carcinogens in Developing Countries

M. Kogevinas, P. Boffetta and N. Pearce

Estimates of exposed populations, prevailing industries and exposures

Precise estimates are not available of the number of workers in developing countries who are exposed to occupational carcinogens. Official statistics on the numbers of workers in specific industries (such as those published by the United Nations) are not fully reliable, since they may not cover major sections of the work-force, such as artisans, small-scale industrial workers and illegal and migrant workers. Further-more, differences in the definition of agricultural workers, who account for a large proportion of the work-force in many developing countries, make international comparisons difficult to interpret. Table 1 gives estimates of the numbers of workers employed in mining, manufacturing and the construction industry in the major developing regions of the world. As might be expected, China accounts for a large proportion of workers in these activities. The very large working populations employed in the construction industry in all regions is noteworthy, as they may have substantial exposure to asbestos.

Table 1. Estimates of working populations in selected activities, by geographical region

Region	Working population (thousands)		
	Mining	Manufacturing	Construction
Latin America	243	14 415	5 451
Middle East and North Africa	157	3 209	1 566
Sub-Saharan Africa	234	2 000	526
China	7 437	32 092	6 023
Asia (excluding China and Middle East)	1 558	24 718	8 000

From United Nations (1987); the estimate refers to 1987 or most recent year available.

An indirect estimate of the number of workers employed in specific industries and of changes in employment patterns with time can be derived from an analysis of patterns and time trends in the production of specific goods. For example, Figure 1 shows the production of asbestos in selected countries in 1973, 1981 and 1990. Countries in southern Africa accounted for about 15% of world production and for 65–70% of production outside of Canada and the former USSR. South Africa is the world's largest producer of amphibole asbestos minerals, and Zimbabwe is the third major producer and supplier of chrysotile asbestos after Canada and the former USSR (Baloyi, 1989). Although production has declined in some developed countries, and in particular Canada, the rapid increase in asbestos production in the USSR and in countries such as Brazil which were not traditional producers is noteworthy. In the same period, the proportion of chrysotile to total asbestos has increased, while the proportion of amphiboles has declined.

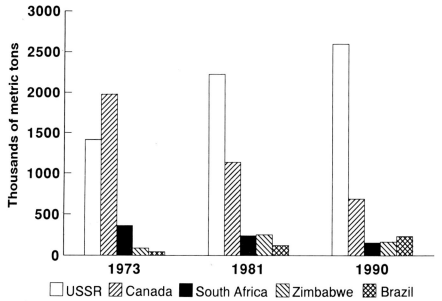

Figure 1. Production of asbestos in selected countries, 1973, 1981 and 1990

From United Nations (1975, 1983); International Asbestos Institute (personal communication)

Figure 2 shows changes in the pattern of tyre production, an industry that may entail increased risks for bladder cancer and leukaemia (see Table 6, Chapter 4). It can be seen that production in developing countries increased rapidly between 1961 and 1987, whereas worldwide production increased by less than 10% between the early and late 1980s (data not shown).

Further information is available from the results of the IARC survey on occupational cancer in developing countries (see Annex 1). Table 2 shows the numbers of workers exposed to asbestos, benzene, nickel and vinyl chloride in countries which responded to the survey questionnaire. Exposure to asbestos was reported in almost

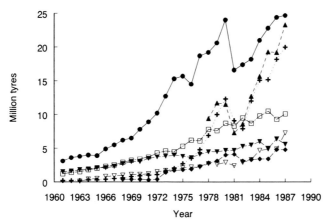

Figure 2. Tyre production in selected countries, 1961–87

From: United Nations (1971, 1987)

●, Brazil; ▲ , China; ▼, India; +, Republic of Korea; □, Mexico; ∇, Turkey

all of the countries and to benzene in many countries, whereas exposure to the other two carcinogens appears to be more sporadic.

Table 3 shows the responses obtained in the same survey with respect to employment in the rubber and chemical industries. With the exception of Peru and Cyprus, both industries are present in all of the countries.

More detailed information on occupational exposures to certain carcinogens is available in some countries. Data on exposures to asbestos, benzene, pesticides and other chemical and physical agents are reviewed in detail below.

Asbestos

Asbestos is the generic name used to describe naturally occurring fibrous minerals of the amphibole and serpentine groups. It is apparently used and handled in all developing and developed countries. Chrysotile (white asbestos), crocidolite (blue asbestos) and amosite (brown asbestos) are the main asbestos minerals exploited commercially. Chrysotile, which accounts for more than 90% of world production, has been mined in Canada, the former USSR and, to a lesser extent, in southern Africa, the USA and Italy. Crocidolite and amosite have been mined mainly in southern Africa (South Africa, Zimbabwe, Swaziland, Mozambique). Overall world production of asbestos decreased in the 1980s, but during the same period the amounts of asbestos mined and consumed in some developing countries increased. The major uses of asbestos are in asbestos–cement products (pipes and building materials), sheets, friction materials, insulation and coating materials and textile products.

Table 2. Numbers of workers exposed to selected occupational carcinogens: results of IARC survey

Country	Asbestos	Benzene	Nickel	Vinyl chloride
Angola	1 000	+		
Bahrain	500−700	1 000−1 500		
Botswana	100	+	200	
Brazil	20−30 000	+		
Chile	+	+		
Cuba	2 200		10 000	
Cyprus	330			
India	9 900			
Jordan	200			
Kuwait	425	235		422
Mongolia				
Morocco	1 300			
Nigeria	+	+	+	+
Peru	600	3 500		100
Philippines	+	+		
Singapore	2 596	1 240		400
Thailand	2 000	4 200		700−900
United Republic of Tanzania	15 600	25 000		15 000
Zimbabwe	+	+		+

+, Exposure occurs, number of exposed workers not known

Table 3. Numbers of workers employed in rubber and chemical industries: results of IARC survey

Country	Rubber industry	Chemical industry
Angola	1 200	+
Bahrain	30	401
Botswana	50	100
Cuba	5 300	10 900
Cyprus		2 800
India	142 000	50 000
Morocco	8 800	24 100
Nigeria	+	+
Philippines	28 000	11 500
Peru		7 860
Thailand	20 000	178 619
United Republic of Tanzania	700	+
Zimbabwe		24 736

+, Employment occurs, number of workers not known

In a series of 68 patients with mesothelioma and a history of occupational exposure in South Africa, 22% had been exposed in the mining industry, 22% on railways, 12% in the construction industry, 10% in the primary asbestos manufacturing industry, 9% in marine engineering and the remainder in other occupations and industries (Solomons, 1984). In a survey of asbestos hazards in developing countries in 1991, responses were received from Botswana, China, Egypt, Honduras, India, Indonesia, Peru, Saudi Arabia, South Africa, Thailand, Turkey and Venezuela. The three leading sources of occupational exposure to asbestos mentioned by respondents were roofing material (in eight), brake linings (in eight), asbestos–cement pipes (in seven), asbestos tiles (in seven), insulation (in three), demolition (in two) and paints, shipyards, filters, a family handicraft industry and installation of home tanks (in one each). The estimated number of workers exposed to asbestos in eight of the countries ranged between 100 to 100 000 (Levy & Seplow, 1992).

In India, 91 440 tonnes of asbestos were estimated to have been used in 1982; 50% of all roofing materials were made from asbestos–cement sheets, and asbestos–cement pipes, used for urban and rural water supplies and sanitation, met about 30% of the country's requirements. Friction materials, bearings, jointings for gaskets, yarns, textiles and asbestos millboard constitute the major non-cement applications of asbestos (Venkataraman, 1982).

Gibbs and du Toit (1973) summarized past measurements of dust concentrations in South African mines and mills. Concentrations in crocidolite mines and mills varied from 2687 particles and fibres per cubic centimetre (p+fpcc) in surface mines in 1940 to 96 p+fpcc in underground mines in 1971. Those in amosite mines and mills were 1458 p+fpcc in surface mines in 1940 and 150 p+fpcc in underground mines in 1971, and those in chrysotile mines and mills were 1734 p+fpcc in surface mines in 1948 and 138 p+fpcc in underground mines in 1971. The authors noted that the data presented were obtained in different locations, using different methods and were usually collected for control rather than epidemiological purposes. The concentrations are, however, based on a sufficient number of samples to represent average levels of exposure.

Zimbabwe is one of the world's major suppliers of chrysotile asbestos and of several important asbestos products. Exposure has been occurring since 1910, when the mines were opened. By 1991, some 7000 men were employed in mines and mills at two sites, Shabanie and Gaths, located some 60 km apart. Another 3000–4000 people were engaged in the manufacture of asbestos construction materials and automotive products (brakes, gaskets, clutches). An undetermined number are exposed in the use, repair and disposal of these materials (Baloyi, 1989; Cullen & Baloyi, 1991; Cullen *et al.*, 1991). Data on the concentrations to which workers have been exposed are, however, scanty. Senior staff at the Sabani and Gath mines estimated that average asbestos concentrations were 30–50 f/ml or more until 1965, and estimated exposures for 1965–80 ranged between 4 and 10 f/ml. Asbestos concentrations have been monitored since 1980 and found to range between 0.5 and 2 f/ml. In an extensive survey conducted in the late 1980s, average concentrations in all job categories at the Sabani mine ranged between 0.1 and 0.27 f/ml, and the actual individual concentrations were

0.01−0.82 f/ml. The respective values for the Gath mine were 0.01−0.28 f/ml and
0.01−0.87 f/ml (Baloyi, 1989).

The Havelock chrysotile mine in Swaziland has been in continuous operation since
the late 1930s. No accurate estimates of past exposure to dust are available, since
monitoring of airborne dust was not started until 1976, when a major dust suppression
programme began. Estimates indicate that levels were extremely high in the past,
particularly in the mill; the airborne dust concentration in an unmanned section at the
time of the report was about 50 f/ml. Employees recalled that in most areas of the mill
the reduction in visibility due to airborne dust was similar to, or worse than, that in
this 'reference' section (McDermott et al., 1982).

A chrysotile mine and mill in Cyprus worked only during the dry season. Dust
concentrations in the mill between 1924 and 1962 (when new mills were built) may
have reached 3000 particles/ml (Gibbs & du Toit, 1973). The concentrations of fibres
longer than 5 μm were 1218 p+fpcc in 1963, 1183 p+fpçc in 1965 and 868 p+fpcc in
1971.

Environmental monitoring was carried out in 1989 in four different mills processing
chrysotile asbestos in the Cuddapah District of Andra Pradesh in India to determine
airborne asbestos fibre levels (Mukherjee et al., 1992). Fibre concentrations in personal
samples and in processing areas were found in most cases to be much higher than the
occupational exposure limits in industrialized countries. Average concentrations in
personal samples were from 1.7 f/ml (range, 1.3−2.1) for workers in the jaw crusher
feeder to 12.9 f/ml (range, 1.8−25.8) for workers in the primary eccentric screen.
Concentrations ranging from 1.9 to 57.7 f/ml were found in short-term personal
samples.

Exposure to asbestos was examined in five asbestos product manufacturing plants
in China which started production in the early 1950s (Wu, 1988). The principal type
of asbestos used was chrysotile. Average dust concentrations between 1956 and 1981,
as determined in 297 samples from five raw material departments, are shown in Figure
3. The asbestos dust levels decreased markedly with time, but even in 1982 average
concentrations greatly exceeded the Chinese standard of 2 mg/m^3.

Exposures to asbestos and the prevalence of asbestosis were investigated in a
chrysotile product factory located in a suburb of Shanghai, China, where asbestos
textile products and friction materials were processed (Huang, 1990). Chinese
chrysotile had been used as the raw material since the factory was founded in 1958,
although Thetford chrysotile asbestos was later imported from Canada. A total of 165
samples were taken at 17 work sites in the factory where asbestos dust was generated.
Average concentrations at 10 work sites within the raw materials preparation
workshop were 2.96 f/ml in braiding and 63.8 f/ml in fibrizing of used material. The
range of individual concentrations was 0.21−177.8 f/ml. Average exposure levels at
four work sites in the fibre workshop ranged from 0.47 to 2.32 f/ml. In the friction
materials workshop, the average dust concentrations ranged from 0.39 to 15.7 f/ml.

Exposure measurements were reported for the period 1964−86 in an asbestos
textile, friction material and cement manufacturing plant in Tianjin, China (Cheng &
Kong, 1992). The factory was set up in 1955 by merging several small asbestos

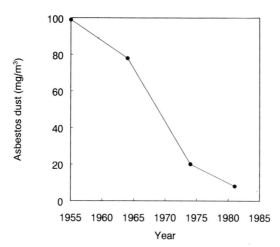

Figure 3. Average concentrations of asbestos dust in five asbestos product plants in China, 1956–81

From Wu (1988)

workshops. The levels of asbestos dust decreased over the measurement period. In the carding and spinning workshop, the highest levels in 1964 were observed in roving (average, 37.5 mg/m^3); the median level in the same department in 1975–86 was 1.2 mg/m^3. In the cement workshop, the highest average levels in 1964 were observed in the mixing operations; the median value in that department in 1975–86 was 20 mg/m^3.

The average annual consumption of crude asbestos in Hong Kong increased from 102 tonnes in 1970–71 to 1107 tonnes in 1978–79, by which time the number of workers estimated to be handling asbestos was about 20 000. The highest exposures occurred in the insulation trade, in shipbuilding and in ship breaking (Lam *et al.*, 1983).

Twelve garages representing the local motor vehicle repair and servicing industry in Hong Kong were surveyed to assess the exposure of workers to asbestos. Chrysotile fibres arising from brake dust and from the machining of asbestos-containing friction material were present in all workshops. The average levels were 0.13 f/ml in personal samples and 0.005 f/ml in static samples (Cheng & O'Kelly 1986).

In a case series of malignant mesotheliomas in Singapore (Ho *et al.*, 1987), two cases occurred in an asbestos product manufacturing factory. The earliest record of air concentrations of asbestos in this factory was from 1981, when they were 0.1–3.9 f/ml.

The importation of asbestos raw materials into the Republic of Korea doubled between 1980 and 1990 when nearly 80 000 tonnes were imported. Most of the imported asbestos material is used in domestic construction and for corrugated cement roof covers; a smaller portion is used in the textile industry. The Republic of Korea supplies asbestos textile and friction products to over 25 countries. The USA and Germany were the biggest importers, but now Japan and many newly developed countries are among the leading importers of asbestos merchandise from the Republic.

An industrial hygiene survey conducted in asbestos textile and slate manufacturing plants showed that the concentrations of asbestos in most plants were 1.3–14.3 f/ml with a geometric mean of 4 f/ml. Forty-nine samples exceeded the national standard of 2 f/ml and 145 samples exceeded the US standard of 0.2 f/ml (Johannig et al., 1991).

An asbestos–cement pipe factory at Mina-Abdulla in Kuwait that began operation in 1977 is the only plant in the country that handles asbestos products (Mohamed, 1990). Chrysotile, crocidolite and amosite asbestos are used. Exposures were measured in 1983 and 1985: the range of asbestos dust was 0.006–0.11 f/ml in 1983 and 0.1–1.65 f/ml in 1985.

Asbestos concentrations were measured in an asbestos–cement factory in Nigeria where both chrysotile and crocidolite were used (Oleru, 1980). Much of the manufacturing process was manual, especially in the mixing of asbestos–cement slurry, removal of the finished product, grinding of pipe joints and ends and transport of asbestos and cement to the mixing area. The concentrations of respirable fibres were correlated with levels of dusty activity in the factory. The highest levels were recorded in the mixing section (6.6 f/ml), with lower levels in the grinding section (4.1 f/ml), and the lowest in the processing section (2.3 f/ml).

Although there are asbestos deposits in Kenya, none is mined and all asbestos is imported. In a study of lung disorders, most cases of asbestosis were identified among workers in a metal factory who were exposed intermittently to asbestos at concentrations below 2 f/ml (Sakari, 1990).

Use of asbestos in Brazil increased dramatically from about 21 500 tonnes in 1967 to about 145 000 tonnes in 1982. Over 80% is in the form of asbestos–cement products, such as roofing tiles and panels, wall-board and domestic and industrial tanks. In a survey of dust concentrations in 1983 in one of the largest asbestos cement plants, in Osasco, most of the 43 samples of inspired air taken at the breathing level contained 0–1.0 f/ml. Peak levels of 3.3 and 4.2 f/ml were observed. Levels were considerably higher in smaller firms (Berman, 1986).

Table 4 provides a summary of studies of exposures to asbestos in various developing countries.

Benzene

Benzene is produced in extremely large quantities worldwide. Occupational exposures occur during the processing of petroleum products, in the coking of coal, during the production of toluene, xylene and other aromatic compounds, in the rubber industry, in consumer products as a chemical intermediate and as a component of gasoline. An association between occupational exposure to benzene and health effects such as aplastic anaemia and leukaemia has been reported in studies of workers in various industries in developing countries, including China, Brazil, Egypt, Myanmar, Nigeria and Turkey, but in many studies levels of exposure were neither measured nor reported. The available results are summarized in Table 5 and described below.

Occupational exposure to benzene was studied in 28 provinces of China between 1970 and 1981. The main source of benzene and mixtures containing benzene was petroleum refineries, but 96% of 528 729 workers in painting, paint production, shoe manufacture, organic synthesis, insulation varnish production, printing industries

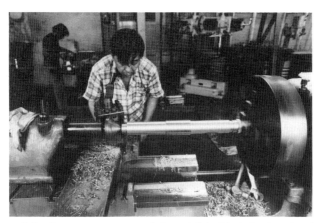

Above: Work with metals leads to exposure not only to metal dust but also to solvents and oils.
Below: Woodworking entails considerable inhalation of solvent vapours and of wood dust containing preservatives
Photos: Courtesy of International Labour Office

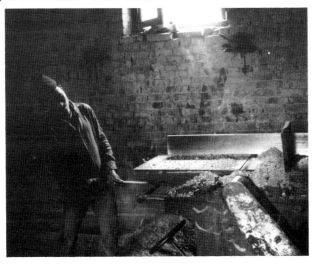

Table 4. Occupational exposure to asbestos fibres in developing countries and regions

Country or region	Occupation/Industry		Exposure level[a]	Comments		Reference
Africa						
Nigeria	Asbestos cement:	mixing	6.6 f/ml	Total respirable fibres,		Oleru (1980)
		milling	4.1 f/ml	chrysotile and crocidolite, circa 1980		
		processing	2.3 f/ml			
Swaziland	Asbestos mill		50 f/ml	1976, chrysotile asbestos, dust, probably representative of past exposure		McDermott et al. (1982)
Zimbabwe	Mining (underground) and milling		30–50 f/ml	Estimated average, chrysotile before 1965 et al. (1991)		Baloyi (1989); Cullen
			4–10 f/ml	Estimated average, chrysotile, 1965–80		
			0.5–2 f/ml	Chrysotile, after 1980		
	Mining (underground) and milling		< 0.01–0.81 f/ml (mean, 0.26)	Bag packer, Shabani mine, chrysotile, early 1980s		Baloyi (1989)
			< 0.14–0.82 f/ml (mean, 0.43)	Floor sweeper, Shabani mine, chrysotile, early 1980s		Baloyi (1989)
			5.55 f/ml	Spill cleaner, Shabani mine, chrysotile, early 1980s		Baloyi (1989)
			0.07–0.87 f/ml (mean, 0.28)	Bag packer, Gaths mine, chrysotile, early 1980s		Baloyi (1989)
South Africa	Surface mining		2687 f+p/cc	1940–45,	crocidolite	Gibbs & du Toit (1973)
			1036 f+p/cc	1950–55,	crocidolite	
			375 f+p/cc	1964–66,	crocidolite	
			273 f+p/cc	1970,	crocidolite	
	Underground mining		1139 f+p/cc	1940–45,	crocidolite	Gibbs & du Toit (1973)
			404 f+p/cc	1950–55,	crocidolite	
			370 f+p/cc	1964–66,	crocidolite	
			146 f+p/cc	1970,	crocidolite	
	Surface mining		1458 f+p/cc	1940–45,	amosite	Gibbs & du Toit (1973)
			646 f+p/cc	1950–55,	amosite	
			495 f+p/cc	1964–66,	amosite	
			354 f+p/cc	1970,	amosite	
	Underground mining		350 f+p/cc	1940–45,	amosite	Gibbs & du Toit (1973)
			445 f+p/cc	1950–55,	amosite	
			150 f+p/cc	1964–66,	amosite	
			150 f+p/cc	1970,	amosite	

Location	Type	Concentration	Description	Fibre type	Reference
South Africa (contd).	Surface mining	1734 f+p/cc	1945–50,	chrysotile	Gibbs & du Toit (1973)
		1684 f+p/cc	1964–66,	chrysotile	
		226 f+p/cc	1970,	chrysotile	
	Underground mining	217 f+p/cc	1945–50,	chrysotile	Gibbs & du Toit (1973)
		196 f+p/cc	1964–66,	chrysotile	
		138 f+p/cc	1970,	chrysotile	
	Surface mining	430 f/ml	1940–45,	long fibres, crocidolite	Gibbs & du Toit (1973)
		6 f/ml	1976–77,	long fibres, crocidolite	
	Underground mining	23 f/ml	1940–45,	long fibres, crocidolite	Gibbs & du Toit (1973)
		2 f/ml	1976–77,	long fibres, crocidolite	
	Surface mining	234 f/ml	1940–45,	long fibres, amosite	Gibbs & du Toit (1973)
		7 f/ml	1976–77,	long fibres, amosite	
	Underground mining	7 f/ml	1940–45,	long fibres, amosite	Gibbs & du Toit (1973)
		3 f/ml	1976–77,	long fibres, amosite	
Asia					
Cyprus	Mining and milling	3000 cc	Estimated, 1924–62		Gibbs & du Toit (1973)
		1218 f+p/cc	Mills, chrysotile, 1963		
		1183 f+p/cc	Mills, chrysotile, 1965		
		868 f+p/cc	Mills, chrysotile, 1971		
Kuwait	Asbestos–cement plant	0.006–0.11 f/ml	Entire indoor working environment, 1983		Mohamed (1990)
		0.1–1.65 f/ml	Entire indoor working environment, 1985		
China, Shanghai	Asbestos product plant	12.6 f/ml (mean)	Raw materials processing		Huang (1990)
		1.4–46.1 f/ml (range)			
		35.7 f/ml (mean)	Grinding		
		7–92.6 f/ml (range)			
		0.8 f/ml (mean)	Weaving fibre		
		0.1–2.3 f/ml (range)			
		15.7 f/ml (mean)	Mixing, friction material		
		2.1–16.3 f/ml (range)			
Rural	Surface mining	46.6–413.0 mg/m^3	Dust crocidolite clay near crushing room, 1984		Liu et al. (1988)
		187.1 mg/ml (mean)			
Rural	Small workplaces	50.1 mg/m^3 (mean)	Four small rural workplaces, 1984		Huang & Zhang (1988)
		265 mg/ml (max.)			
Tianjin	Asbestos textile	22.5 mg/m^3 (mean)	Concentration of asbestos dust, cording and spinning, milling, 1964		Cheng & Kong (1992)
		16.7 mg/m^3 (mean)	As above, milling, 1974		

Country or region	Occupation/Industry	Exposure level[a]	Comments	Reference
China (contd). Tianjin (contd).	Asbestos textile (contd)	14.7 mg/m^3 (median)	As above, milling, 1978–86	Cheng & Kong (1992)
		34.5 mg/m^3 (mean)	As above, mixing, 1964	
		12.7 mg/m^3 (median)	As above, mixing, 1974	
		10.2 mg/m^3 (mean)	As above, mixing, 1975–86	
		12.6 mg/m^3 (mean)	Concentration of asbestos dust, twisting, universal winding, 1964	
	Friction material	3.2 mg/m^3 (mean)	As above, winding, 1974	
		2.4 mg/m^3 (median)	As above, winding, 1975–86	
		8.3 mg/m^3 (mean)	As above, braiding, 1964	
		3.8 mg/m^3 (mean)	As above, braiding, 1974	
		2.3 mg/m^3 (median)	As above, braiding, 1975–86	
		22.5 mg/m^3 (mean)	Grinding, 1964	
		24.3 mg/m^3 (mean)	Grinding, 1974	
		3.8 mg/m^3 (median)	Grinding, 1975–86	
		20.2 mg/m^3 (mean	Mixing, 1974	
		10.5 (median)	Mixing, 1975–86	
		88.8 mg/m^3 (mean)	Crushing, 1974	
		2.8 mg/m^3 (median)	Crushing, 1975–86	
	Asbestos–cement	41.4 mg/m^3 (mean)	Milling, 1964	
		23.8 mg/m^3 (mean)	Milling, 1974	
		20.8 mg/m^3 (median)	Milling, 1975–86	
		34.2 mg/m^3 (mean)	Crushing, 1964	
		24.2 mg/m^3 (mean)	Crushing, 1974	
		14.6 mg/m^3 (median)	Crushing, 1975–86	
		166.6 mg/m^3 (mean)	Mixing, 1964	
		39.6 mg/m^3 (mean)	Mixing, 1974	
		20.0 mg/m^3 (median)	Mixing, 1975–86	
Various areas	Asbestos product manufacturers	About 100 mg/m^3	Average in five raw materials departments, around 1955	Wu (1988)
		About 80 mg/m^3	As above, around 1965	
		About 20 mg/m^3	As above, around 1975	
		About 10 mg/m^3	As above, around 1982	
Hong Kong	Motor vehicle repair and servicing	0.01–0.83 f/ml (mean, 0.13) 0.0–0.54 f/ml	Personal sample, around 1985	Cheng & O'Kelly (1986)
		(mean, 0.05)	Static sample, around 1985	

Region	Industry/process	Concentration	Notes	Reference
Republic of Korea	Asbestos textile	1.3–14.3 f/ml (geometric mean, 4.4)	All samples > 0.4 f/ml; 49 samples > 2 f/ml, chrysotile, 1987	Johannig et al. (1991)
Singapore	Asbestos–cement plant	0.1–3.9 f/ml	Mixed asbestos fibres, highest value in mixing department, 1981	Ho et al. (1987)
	Asbestos product manufacturing factory	0.1–3.9 g/ml	Air concentrations, 1981	Ho et al. (1987)
India	Mining	< 1 f/ml	1977–90	Indian National Institute of Occupational Health (1989–90)
	Milling	4–488 f/ml	1977–90	
Andhra Pradesh	Chrysotile milling	4.8 f/ml (mean); 2.2–8.2 f/ml (range)	Jaw crusher, 1989, short-term sample, 60–100 cm from process	Mukherjee et al. (1992)
		29.1 f/ml (mean); 16.5–41.6 f/ml (range)	Pulverizer, as above	
		9.3 f/ml (mean); 1.9–23.4 f/ml (range)	Lime-mix, as above	
		17.1 f/ml (mean); 11.4–22.3 f/ml (range)	Huller feeder, as above	
		15.6 f/ml (mean); 8.2–26.4 f/ml (range)	Primary eccentric screen, as above	
		22.4 f/ml (mean); 4.3–57.5 f/ml (range)	Decorticator, as above	
		1.7 f/ml (mean); 1.3–2.1 f/ml (range)	Jaw crusher feeder, 1989; personal samples, 15–60 min	
		8.9 f/ml (mean); 2.3–15.4 f/ml (range)	Pulverizer, as above	
		2.6 f/ml (mean); 2.5–2.6 f/ml (range)	Lime-mix, as above	
		12.7 f/ml (mean); 8.9–16.4 f/ml (range)	Huller feeder, as above	
		12.9 f/ml (mean); 1.8–25.8 f/ml (range)	Primary eccentric screen, as above	
		8.8 f/ml (mean); 1.3–18.4 f/ml (range)	Decorticator, as above	
South America				
Brazil	Asbestos–cement plant	0.0–1.0 f/ml (range); 4.2 f/ml (max).	Majority of samples, breathing zone, 1983	Berman (1986)

f/ml, fibres per millilitre; f+p/cc, fibres and particles per cubic centimetre

Table 5. Occupational exposure to benzene in developing countries

Country	Occupation/Industry	Exposure level	Comments	Reference
Africa				
Egypt	Rubber coating plants	5.4 ppm (mean)	Mixing, area samples, plant A	Noweir (1986)
		0–12 ppm (range)		
		10.5 ppm (mean)	Mixing, area samples, plant B	
		0.5–20.5 ppm (range)		
		7.2 ppm (mean)	Coating, sampling near	
		1–13.5 ppm (range)	machines, plant A	
		12.9 ppm (mean)	Coating, sampling near	
		2.5–23.0 ppm (range)	machines, plant B	
Asia				
Turkey	Shoemakers	15–30 ppm	Outside working hours, around 1970	Aksoy et al. (1974)
		210 ppm (max.)	When adhesive applied	
India	Petrol pump attendants	1.43 ppm (mean)	Breathing zone samples, 1991	Das et al. (1991)
Myanmar	Petrol pump attendants	61.9 mg/L (mean)	Urinary phenol content, around 1985	Hein et al. (1989)
		17–320 mg/L		
China	Many plants	0.06–849.7 mg/m^3	Paint workers, chemical synthesis,	Yin et al. (1987)
		(95% range)	insulation varnish production,	
		18.1 mg/cm^3 (geometric mean)	shoemaking, etc., 1979–81	
South America				
Brazil	Steel workers	300–1000 ppm/day	Exposure during frequent accidents	S. Barreto (personal
			in coke oven and by-products plant	communication)
	Shoemakers	6.5 mg/g creatinine	Urinary phenol, 79 factory workers,	de Fernicola et al.
			São Paulo, around 1975	(1976)
		4.2 mg/g creatinine	Urinary phenol, 65 domestic	
			shoeworkers, around 1975	
	Petrochemical	44 ppm (upper limit)	Personal samples during change	Kato et al. (1993)
			of packs, maintenance of	
			equipment containing chemicals	
		1.5–6.5 ppm	Area samples in unit using benzene as solvent	
		0.05–2 ppm	Area samples in unit using benzene as raw material	

and rubber refineries were studied. Of these, 26 319 in 50 255 workplaces were exposed to benzene and the rest to mixtures containing benzene. The benzene concentration in 65% of the workplaces was less than 40 mg/m^3; concentrations in excess of 1000 mg/m^3 were found in 1.3% of the workplaces (Figure 4). The geometric mean concentration of benzene was 18.1 mg/m^3 (95% confidence interval, 0.06–849.7). The prevalence of poisoning was 0.94% among workers exposed to benzene and 0.44% among those exposed to mixtures. In a shoe-making plant in which four cases of aplastic anaemia cases were observed, a 1:3 mixture of chlorobutadiene and benzene was used, and the average daily concentration of benzene was estimated to be 1036 mg/m^3 (Yin *et al.*, 1987).

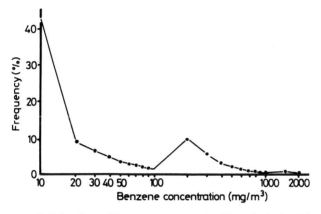

Figure 4. Frequency distribution of benzene concentrations in industries in 28 counties in China

From Yin *et al.* (1987)

An occupational health survey was conducted on workers who inhale petrol fumes containing low concentrations of benzene at petrol filling stations in the city of Rangoon, Myanmar. Exposure was evaluated by measuring urinary phenol concentrations for the workers and for a healthy control group. The average urinary phenol concentration among petrol filling station workers was 61.9 mg/L (range, 17–320) (Hein *et al.*, 1989).

Aksoy and his colleagues (1974) examined exposure to benzene and other solvents and the occurrence of leukaemia and other haematological disorders among shoemakers in Istanbul, Turkey. The concentration of benzene in the work environment was reported to range between 15 and 30 ppm outside working hours but to rise to 210 ppm when adhesives containing benzene were used. Peak exposures of 210 and 650 ppm were recorded in small, poorly ventilated areas. The benzene concentration in the air of a tyre cord manufacturing factory where two cases of acute leukaemia were recorded over a six-year period was 110 ppm (Aksoy *et al.*, 1987).

In São Paulo, Brazil, average urinary phenol concentrations were 6.5 mg/g creatinine in 79 shoe factory workers and 4.2 ng/g creatinine in 65 workers making shoes at home (de Fernicola *et al.*, 1976). Faria (1987) reported levels of 1000, 2000 and

2533 ppm benzene in different sectors of the metal industry in the Cubatao region of Brazil.

The Camaçari Petrochemical Complex is the largest, most important industrial complex in north-eastern Brazil, employing about 50 000 workers. Benzene and its homologues, n-hexane, haloalkanes and some alcohols were used extensively as solvents or raw materials. The highest levels of benzene were recorded during maintenance of equipment containing chemicals, and personal air sampling during changing of packs indicated levels as high as 44 ppm. Concentrations of 1.5−6.5 ppm were found in a unit where benzene was used as a solvent and lower levels (0.05−2.0 ppm) in a unit where it was used as a raw material (Kato et al., 1993).

Average exposures to benzene in mixing areas in rubber coating plants in Egypt ranged between 5.4 and 10.5 ppm. Area samples taken near the coating machines contained average concentrations of 7.2−12.9 ppm (Noweir, 1986).

Pesticides

The use of pesticides has increased dramatically in both industrialized and developing countries during the few last decades, predominantly for use in agriculture, horticulture and vector control. Significant amounts are also used in forestry and livestock production. In public health, pesticides are used mainly to control five vector-borne diseases: malaria, filariasis, onchocerciasis, schistosomiasis and trypano-somiasis (Edwards, 1986). An estimated 50 000 tonnes of pesticides were used for public health problems in developing countries in 1980, accounting for about 10% of worldwide pesticide use. The absence of measurements of long-term occupational exposure to pesticides in developing countries is, however, striking.

World sales of pesticides used in agriculture and in the control of disease vectors increased from US$ 8.1 billion in 1972 to 12.8 billion in 1983, in adjusted dollars (World Resources Institute, 1986). The most rapid growth in use was observed in developing countries, where the cost of importation of various chemicals rose 6.5 fold during the period 1970−80. It is estimated that about 20% of the world's agrochemicals are used in developing countries. Pesticide sales during 1983−87 in the Philippines, a country where pesticides are used heavily in selected regions (Loevinsohn, 1987), are shown in Figure 5. A dramatic increase in the importation and use of pesticides was reported in Kenya in the late 1980s (Figure 6).

DDT was one of the first pesticides to be used widely in both industrialized and developing countries, but its use has been severely restricted or banned in many industrialized countries since the early 1970s. DDT was introduced in India for use in public health and agriculture in 1948. Since then, nearly 250 000 tonnes have been used, 50 000 tonnes of which in agriculture. Use of DDT in India over the period 1960−84 is shown in Figure 7; its use for agricultural purposes was banned in 1989. In Iraq, about 12 000 tonnes of DDT were used by the agricultural authorities between 1960 and 1978. In Pakistan, the yearly agricultural use of DDT (as the active ingredient) during the period 1977−81 ranged from 40 to 100 tonnes. In one province in Indonesia, a large-scale malaria control programme was begun in 1952, and between 1952 and 1980 as much as 1400 tonnes of DDT were used annually (IARC, 1991).

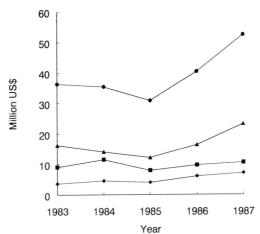

Figure 5. Pesticide sales in the Philippines on the basis of total imports, 1983–87

From Lum *et al.* (1993). ●, all pesticides; ▲, insecticides, ◆, herbicides; ■, fungicides

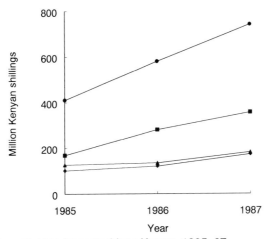

Figure 6. Values of pesticides imported into Kenya, 1985–87

From Mwanthi and Kimani (1993). ●, all pesticides; ▲, insecticides; ◆, herbicides; ■, fungicides

Pesticides have become an important export commodity: the world export value of pesticide products nearly tripled during the period 1970–87, rising to almost US$ 6000 million. A considerable proportion of the pesticides that are exported from industrialized countries to developing countries are products that are banned or severely restricted in industrialized countries (see also Chapter 2). It is difficult to obtain an accurate picture of pesticide exports to developing countries because descriptions of the exported pesticide products and the companies shipping them are frequently missing

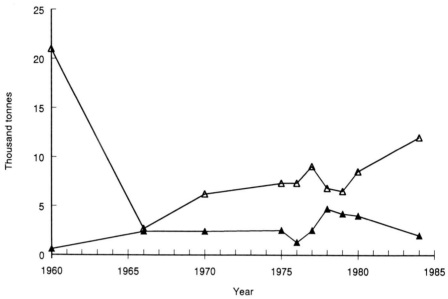

Figure 7. Use of DDT in India, 1960–84

From IARC (1991). △, public health; ▲ , agriculture

or incomplete. Of the nearly 228 million kg of pesticides exported from the USA in 1991, 58.3% were identified only by general terms or by trade names that cannot be found in standard reference books on pesticide production (Foundation for Advancements in Science and Education, 1993); an additional 16.2% are identified only by chemical family name or by an incomplete chemical name. No information is therefore available on about 75% of all chemicals exported from the USA. It has been estimated, however, that in 1991 at least 1.9 million kg of pesticides that are banned, cancelled or voluntarily suspended in the USA were exported, including 97.5 tonnes of DDT. Large quantities of pesticides that are unregistered (and therefore not used) in the USA were also exported, including butachlor (4 572 000 tonnes exported to Argentina, Belgium, China, Colombia, India, Japan, the Philippines and Thailand) and ethylene dibromide (855 000 tonnes exported mainly to South Africa). About 3 million kg of chlordane, heptachlor and carbofuran, which are severely restricted pesticides in the USA, were exported to Third World countries in 1991 (Foundation for Advancements in Science and Education, 1993).

Numerous reports have been made of acute intoxication from pesticides, and various estimates have been reported of fatalities. Although peak exposures (such as those that provoke acute intoxications) cannot be used to estimate long-term occupational exposures, they provide an unequivocal picture of the lack of hygiene measures in the handling of pesticides. It has been estimated that 99% of all deaths due to acute pesticide poisoning occur in developing countries, where, however, only 20% of the world's agrochemicals are used. Several estimates have been made of the extent of acute pesticide poisoning at a global level, which were summarized by Jeyaratnam (1992):

> Our picture of the extent of acute poisoning on a global scale is largely based, of necessity, on estimates. The first such estimate was done by the World Health Organization (1973), which suggested that 500 000 cases of pesticide poisoning occurred annually. At that time it was considered to be an unacceptably large problem, requiring efforts to substantiate this estimate as well as to control the problem.
>
> ... The magnitude of the global problem of acute pesticide poisoning was further heightened by an estimate in 1985 (Jeyaratnam, 1985a) of approximately three million cases hospitalized annually, resulting in approximately 220 000 deaths.
>
> In 1986, the WHO made an estimate of one million cases of unintentional pesticide poisoning resulting in 20 000 deaths, which is in harmony with the earlier estimates of Jeyaratnam (1985b), as approximately two-thirds of the cases of acute pesticide poisoning are thought to be due to suicidal intent ....

Studies in South-East Asia indicate that suicide is the major cause of pesticide-related acute deaths; however, in other regions, for example Latin America, occupational exposures appear to be the major cause. In Costa Rica, 6.4% of pesticide poisonings were estimated to be suicides and 67.8% due occupational exposures (Forget, 1991).

Few quantitative data are available on levels of exposure of workers to pesticides in developing countries. Selected studies in which occupational exposures in production, spraying and application of pesticides were reported are shown in Table 6.

Studies of the use of protective clothing by pesticide sprayers and applicators in developing countries indicate that most workers do not use such protection, which is designed for colder climates — made of plastic or rubber material — and may thus cause considerable discomfort when worn in hot, humid climates. In Malaysia, as in many other countries, the application techniques used increase the exposure of pesticide applicators. Thus, foliage is sprayed mainly using knapsack sprayers designed 30–40 years ago (Lum *et al.*, 1993). In a survey of 27 Malaysian plantation workers spraying paraquat, 15 workers used no protection and nine used only limited protection (boots or gloves). Sprayers showered regularly after work and changed their clothes but rarely bothered to wash off minor splashes and washed only infrequently before eating when at work (Howard *et al.*, 1981).

In a study in Bolivia on pesticide poisoning among 534 agricultural workers exposed directly to pesticides, of 131 workers in the lowlands, 69% used no personal protection and 92% bathed after spraying. Of 403 workers in the uplands and other regions, 93% wore no personal protection, and 26% bathed after spraying (Condarco Aguilar *et al.*, 1993). In a large study in the rural township of Carmen de Viboral, Colombia, 5483 subjects were interviewed concerning the use of paraquat: 94.5% of the paraquat users applied the herbicide with sprayers. Of those, 76% considered their spraying equipment to be in good condition, and 71% reported that paraquat wet their bodies

Table 6. Occupational exposures to pesticides in developing countries

Pesticide	Population	Levels[a]	Reference
Cypermethrin	Applicators treating crops in the United Republic of Tanzania, the Ivory Coast and Paraguay using an Electrodynsprayer	3.0–26.9 mg/h (D) (total contamination)	Dover (1985)
	Applicators treating crops in the United Republic of Tanzania and the Ivory Coast using a spinning disc sprayer	17.8–369.9 mg/h (D) (total contamination)	
	Applicators treating crops in Paraguay using a knapsack sprayer	29.5 mg/h (D) (total contamination)	
Dimethoate	Eight spraymen using a knapsack sprayer for treatment of crops in the Sudan	Total calculated exposure: 175.8 µg–8.3 mg/cm² per day (D); 5.1–19.9 mg/day (R)	Copplestone et al. (1976)
Pyrethroid formulation	Seven applicators spraying cotton in the Ivory Coast	Total exposure: 2.8–42.2 mg/h (D); < 100–200 mg/m³ (R)	Prinsen & Van Sittert (1980)
Malathion	Spraymen treating interior household surfaces for mosquito control in Pakistan	300 mg (average daily dermal exposure)	Baker et al. (1978)
Pyrethroids	199 production workers in dividing and packaging, China, 1983–84	0.012–0.055 mg/m³, air concentration, fenvalerate; 0.005–0.012 mg/m³, air concentration, deltamethrin; 1.02–18.6 mg/L, urine concentration, fenvalerate	He et al. (1988)

[a] D, dust sample; R, respirator sample

during spraying. It was generally considered that safety instructions were not followed properly in the region (Arroyave, 1993).

In the Jordan Valley of the West Bank, spraying of crops with pesticides has increased tremendously over the last 20 years. In a survey of 79 sprayers of organophosphates in the region, only 4% wore protective clothing, and 92% had ever spilt pesticides on their body; 88% changed clothes after spraying, 25% bathed after spraying, and 33% reported unusual symptoms after spraying (Sansur *et al.*, 1993).

Exposures to other organic chemicals

Studies of exposures to other organic chemicals are summarized in Table 7.

Exposures to *vinyl chloride monomer* ranging between 1000 and 10 000 ppm were reported in a Malaysian electrochemical factory near vats where polyvinyl chloride was produced. Concentrations up to 100 ppm were reported in vats at the time workers entered to clean them (Ives, 1986).

Wu (1988) reported levels of exposure to *vinyl chloride monomer* in 14 major production facilities in China during 1958–81. Concentrations were very high prior to 1970. Control measures were adopted after 1970, but the levels of exposure continued to be high because operations were carried out manually in many sites within the plants. Average levels in the first compressor room were 469 ppm in 1978 and 222 ppm in 1981; the levels in all other departments were considerably lower.

Exposure to *vinyl chloride* was examined in a shoe factory in Nigeria where polyvinyl chloride pellets were heated with additives and plasticizers and stabilizers were fed into ducts connected to moulds in which footwear was shaped upon cooling. The main source of exposure to vinyl chloride was probably at the moulds. The average concentration of vinyl chloride recorded at the factory was 1.6 ppm (range, 0–4.0; eight samples) (Oleru & Onyekwere, 1992).

In *benzidine* production and use facilities in Tianjin, Shanghai and Jilin, China, the production of direct dyes was based on imported powdered benzidine base and benzidine hydrochloride until about 1956, when production of benzidine begun in Tianjin and Jilin. More than 100 000 tonnes of benzidine were produced between 1956 and 1977, when production ceased. Benzidine concentrations were measured in the ambient air in Tianjin and Jilin during 1962–70, and skin contamination and urine concentrations of benzidine were determined for selected workers in Tianjin. Average ambient air levels ranged from 0.05 to 0.39 mg/m^3 and were highest near pressure filters and lower in transformation areas. Average concentrations on hands and skin were 3.3–11.7 $\mu g/m^3$, while urinary benzidine concentrations ranged from non-detectable levels to 0.77 mg/24 h (Bi *et al.*, 1992).

Urine samples from workers in a small-scale unit for the manufacture of Direct Black 38 in India were analysed by high-pressure liquid chromatography for the presence of *benzidine* and mono- and diacetyl benzidine (Dewan *et al.*, 1988). Acetylated metabolites were found in all 18 urine samples, and benzidine was found in all except two (average, 48.2 $\mu g/L$; range, 0–362.5).

Levels of *benzo[a]pyrene* were measured in a shale-oil production plant in China, built in the 1920s (Wu, 1988). Data obtained in 1975 indicated that air concentrations

Table 7. Occupational exposures to various organic chemicals in developing countries

Country	Occupation/Industry	Exposure	Comments	Reference
Nigeria	Shoe factory	**Vinyl chloride** 1.6 ppm (mean) 0–4.0 ppm (range)	Plastics section, 8 samples	Oleru & Onyekwere (1992)
China	14 production facilities	1.8 ppm (mean) 0.5–214 ppm (range) 77 ppm (mean) 14–367 ppm (range) 469 ppm (mean) 144–4600 ppm (range) 222 ppm (mean) 41–1540 ppm (range) 85 ppm (mean) 4–4900 ppm (range) 61 ppm (mean) 9–244 ppm (range) 25 ppm (mean) 1–163 ppm (range) 9 ppm (mean) 4–145 ppm (range) 5 ppm (mean) 1–18 ppm (range)	Synthetic control room, 13 samples, 1978 Synthetic room at building, 13 samples, 1978 Compressor room 1, 12 samples, 1978 Compressor room 1, 23 samples, 1981 Compressor room 2, 12 samples, 1978 Polymerizing room, 13 samples, 1978 Polymerizing room, 23 samples, 1981 Basic processing, 10 samples, 1978 Packing, 12 samples, 1978	Wu (1988)
China	Dye production	**Benzidine** (mean) 0.05 mg/m^3 (high) 0.9 mg/m^3 (mean) 0.24 mg/cm^3 (mean) 0.16 mg/cm^3 (mean) 0.39 mg/cm^3 (mean) 0.27 mg/cm^3	Transformation area, 1962 Filtration area, 1962 Oil pump, 1962 Packaging, 1965 Underground tub, 1970	Bi et al. (1992)
India	Dye production	260.3 mg/L 362.5 mg/L	Benzidine in urine, production of Direct Black 38, highest levels detected around 1985	Dewan et al. (1988)
China	Anatomists	**Formaldehyde** 2–3 mg/m^3	Highest level in breathing zone, around 1980	Zhang & Jiang (1988)

in the plant were between 2 and 12.4 µg/100 m^3. The concentration on top of an oven in one department was 33.7 µg/100 m^3.

Most plants in China where *chloromethyl methyl ether* and bis(chloromethyl) ether are produced were built between the late 1950s and the early 1970s. In one plant in Shanghai, the concentrations of chloromethyl methyl ether in 1977–78 were 1.2–59 ppm, but they may have been higher prior to 1977 (Wu, 1988).

Air *pitch* concentrations in two carbon producing plants, built in China in the 1950s, were 40 mg/m^3, although air contamination at work sites during the early years of operation was reported to have been extraordinarily severe (Wu, 1988).

Exposures to dust

Evidence of exposure to *dust* (other than asbestos) in mines and certain workplaces comes from many sources; these studies are summarized in Table 8. The prevalence of silicosis among miners and other workers has been studied in many countries (see chapter 8), but dust concentrations were not measured or not reported in most. Noweir (1986) reported high prevalences of silicosis among workers in various industries in Egypt: 43% among 605 workers in phosphate mining; 25% of 1292 workers in two haematite mines (including crushing); 33% in two plants for the manufacture of refractory materials employing 1197 workers. High prevalences of silicosis were also observed among workers in steel mills (preparation of ore), china and ceramics manufacture and foundries. While dust levels in these industries must have been high, no measurements were reported.

A study in a large coal mine in eastern China reported *dust* concentrations during different methods of drilling and with various ventilation systems. Average dust concentrations were above 20 mg/m^3 for dry drilling with poor ventilation; when a wet drilling system and improved ventilation were used, 95% of measurements showed concentrations below 2 mg/m^3. In 1953, average dust concentrations were reported to be as high as 266 mg/m^3 (Yang *et al.*, 1985).

Studies were conducted in various areas in China of workers in tungsten, copper–iron and tin mines and pottery workers in relation to exposure to *dust*, to radon decay products and to various metals (Chen *et al.*, 1992; McLaughlin *et al.*, 1992; Laurer *et al.*, 1993). The average annual dust levels by type of facility were 6.1 mg/m^3 (range, 2.0–26.43) in tungsten mines, 5.6 mg/m^3 (range, 3.8–16.1) in copper–iron mines and 7.7 mg/m^3 (range, 3.4–29.7) in tin mines.

A high prevalence of silicosis was observed among workers in the Anshan Iron and Steel Company in China, which started operating in 1951 (Goldsmith, 1985). In 1983, 21% of air dust measurements at 129 inspection stations showed concentrations of silica above the standard of 10 mg/m^3.

Dust concentrations were measured for 26 603 workers in two metallic mines (one lead, one molybdenum), two coal mines, a fireproof raw materials workshop in a steel plant, a foundry in a large machinery plant and a raw material workshop in a glass factory in China (Lou & Zhou, 1989). Average dust concentrations decreased sharply after installation of wet mining and engineering control methods. Before the control measures were taken, the highest average levels were observed in the lead mine (340 mg/m^3, 31.5% SiO$_2$); after installation of controls, the highest levels were

Table 8. Occupational exposures to dust in mining and other industries in developing countries

Country	Occupation/Industry	Exposure level	Comments	Reference
Africa				
Kenya	Mining, quarrying, calcining of diatomaceous earth	0.7 mg/m³ 3.8 mg/m³	Laboratory workers Bag filling, packaging	Sakari (1990)
South Africa	Ceramics industry	0.33 mg/m³ (median)	Repirable quartz dust; production in pottery industry, 1973–86, 7 samples	Rees & Kielkowski (1991)
		0.16–0.40 m/gm³ (range)	As above; manufacturing, 20 samples	
		0.04 mg/m³ (median)	Respirable quartz; basic plant,	
		0–0.07 mg/m³ (range)	refractory industry, 1973–86, 6 samples	
		0.13 mg/m³ (median)	As above; acid plant, 9 samples	
		0.04–0.43 mg/m³ (range)		
	Lapidary industry (precious stones)	< 0.0001 mg/m³	Cape Town, respirable dust level, 79–81% free crystalline silica, late 1980	White et al. (1991)
Asia				
China	Coal mine	> 20 mg/m³	Dry drilling, poor ventilation, average of 36 samples, 1980s	Yang et al. (1985)
		> 5 mg/m³	Wet drilling, improved ventilation, 1980s; 3 samples	
		2–5 mg/m³	As above; 18 samples	
		< 2 mg/m³	As above; 36 samples	
		266 mg/m³	Underground dust concentrations, 1953	
	Lead mine	340 mg/m³ (mean)	Average dust concentrations, 31.5% SiO₂; 18 samples, 1956	Lou & Zhou (1989)
		5.7 mg/m³ (mean)	As above; 2038 samples, 1957–81	
	Molybdenum mine	315 mg/m³ (mean)	As above; 5.0% SiO₂; 24 samples, 1956	
		4.7 mg/m³ (mean)	As above; 43 621 samples, 1957–81	
	Coal mines	217 mg/m³ (mean)	As above; 27% SiO₂, 49 samples, 1960–62	
		17.3 mg/m³ (mean)	As above; 6888 samples, 1963–81	
	Machinery plant	201 mg/m³ (mean)	Foundry, 85–97% SiO₂; 111 samples, 1956–62	
		29.3 mg/m³ (mean)	As above; 144 samples, 1963–81	
South America				
Chile	Copper mine	189.5 mg/m³ (mean)	10 samples; respirable silica dust (mostly crystalline) among workers in crushing plant	Romo-Kroger et al. (1989)

observed in the cast steel company (29.3 mg/m^3) and the two coal mines (17.2 and 17.8 mg/m^3).

In a study in Kenya, 27 of 54 workers involved in the quarrying, drying/calcining, packaging and storage of diatomaceous earth were found to have silicosis at various stages. *Dust* concentrations varied between 0.17 mg/m^3 in the laboratory to 3.8 mg/m^3 in bag filling and packaging. Respirable dust contained an average of 6.9% crystalline silica (Sakari, 1990).

Exposure to quartz *dust* was examined among workers in coffee processing factories in Uganda. At harvest time, coffee (and cotton) are dried on the ground, which is usually soil. By the time the crop reaches the coffee hulling factories, it is loaded with appreciable amounts of respirable soil *dust*, and the pre-cleaning sections of such factories are laden with both organic and inorganic dust. A study in 22 coffee processing factories in Uganda in 1989 indicated that the respirable dust in pre-cleaning sections contained 40−60% quartz dust by weight, corresponding in terms of concentration to over 0.2 mg/m^3 of quartz (Ogaram, 1990).

Rees and Kielkowski (1991) examined *dust* levels in three ceramics factories in South Africa between 1973 and 1987. In a pottery industry, median respirable quartz concentrations were highest in the production section (0.33 mg/m^3). In a refractory ceramics plant, the median levels of respirable quartz were highest in the acid plant (0.13 mg/m^3). Concentrations of respirable quartz were not available for the brickworks factory, but 126 samples out of a total of 268 contained levels of respirable dust above 2 mg/m^3.

Exposure to respirable *dust* among gemstone workers was evaluated in Cape Town, South Africa, to be below 0.0001 mg/m^3. The free crystalline content of samples was 79−81% (White *et al.*, 1991).

Exposure to silica *dust* was examined among workers in the crushing plant of a copper mine in Chile (Romo-Kroger *et al.*, 1989). In 10 samples of particulate matter collected in the respiratory protection equipment used by the workers, the concentration of silica (mostly crystalline silica) was 0.19 mg/m^3.

Exposures to metals

Studies of exposure to metals are summarized in Table 9.

Hair samples from mine workers in Obuasi, Ghana, were examined in order to assess the degree of exposure to *arsenic*. Samples from those working in roaster and chemical processing sections showed a high content of 1013 ppm by weight (Amasa, 1975).

The highest urinary concentrations of *arsenic* among workers in a copper, arsenic, gold and silver mine complex in Chile in the 1980s were found among packers (0.17 µg/L) (Harper & Possel Miranda, 1990).

Exposure to *arsenic* was estimated in four tin mines in Yunnan Province, China (Sun, 1988; Qiao *et al.*, 1989; Taylor *et al.*, 1989). Airborne dust concentrations, first measured in the 1950s when dry drilling was common, reached 20−102.6 mg/m^3; they fell appreciably after 1964 when wet drilling became widespread. Arsenic represented 1.34% of the mined ore by weight as As$_2$O$_3$. The mean arsenic content of airborne dust was 0.42 mg/m^3 before 1952; direct measurements of arsenic in air conducted in the

M. *Kogevinas et al.*

Table 9. Occupational exposures to metals in developing countries

Country	Occupation/Industry	Exposure	Comments	Reference
Africa		**Arsenic**		
Ghana	Gold mine	44 ppm	Content by weight in hair samples; 8 mine workers in shaft	Amasa (1975)
		1013 ppm	As above; 7 workers in roaster and chemical processing sectors	
Asia				
China	Tin mine	0.42 mg/m^3 (mean)	Air measurements, 1952	Qiao *et al.* (1989)
		0.01 mg/m^3 (mean)	As above, 1980s	
South America				
Chile	Copper, arsenic, gold and silver mine complex	0.065 mg/L (mean)	Urinary concentration, 1980s; grill workers	Harper & Possel Miranda (1990)
		0.125 mg/L (mean)	As above, roaster operators	
		0.17 mg/L (mean)	As above, packers	
Asia		**Cadmium**		
China	Cadmium refining, Hunan Province	0.074 mg/m^3	Concentration of cadmium oxide in foundry, 1973	Liu *et al.* (1985)
		0.13 mg/m^3	As above, 1978	
		0.004−0.187 mg/m^3	Average air concentrations in breathing zone of operators in various departments, 1982	
		5.03 mg/g creatinine (mean)	Levels in urine of 65 workers, 1982	
		0.90−79.00 mg/g creatinine (range)		
		20.4 mg/L (mean)	Levels in blood of 65 workers, 1982	
		1.00−92.5 mg/L (range)		
	Tin mine, Yunnan Province	< 0.05 mg/m^3 (mean)	Air measurements in mine, 1977	Taylor *et al.* (1989)

Table 9 (contd)

Country	Occupation/Industry	Exposure	Comments	Reference
Singapore	Storage battery factory	0.39 mg/m³ (geometric mean)	Air, tablet-making process, 5 samples, 1980	Chen *et al.* (1982)
		0.87 mg/m³ (geometric mean)	As above, spot welding, 5 samples, 1980	
		154.6 mg/L (geometric mean)	Blood, spot welders, 10 measurements, 1980	
		58.3 mg/L (geometric mean)	As above, tablet-makers, plate-forming workers, 31 measurements, 1980	
		0.64 mg/m³ (geometric mean)	Workroom air, 5 static samples, 1976	
		0.13 mg/m³ (geometric mean)	As above, 3 samples, 1978	
South America				
Brazil	Motor vehicle battery repair, Salvador, Bahia	0.07 mmol/L (geometric mean) 0.004–0.247 nmol/L (range)	Blood levels, 39 samples, 1980s	Carvalho *et al.* (1985)
Asia		**Chromates**		
China	Chromate production, seven cities	0.02–21.3 mg/m³	Air levels; range of exposures between 1963 and 1980. Exposure believed to be much higher occasionally	Wu (1988)
	Tin mine, Yunnan Province	0.55 mg/m³	Mean air measurements in mine, 1977	Taylor *et al.* (1989)

1980s showed a considerably lower mean concentration of 0.01 mg/m^3. Several other minerals also present in the ore were measured: air samples taken in 1977 showed mean values of less than 0.05 µg/m^3 for cadmium, 0.075 µg/m^3 for nickel and 0.55 µg/m^3 for chromium (Taylor et al., 1989).

The extent of exposure to *cadmium* was studied in workers in a cadmium—nickel battery factory in Singapore (Chen et al., 1982). Air, blood and urinary cadmium levels were particularly high in the workers. In 1980, the highest levels were associated with spot welding (geometric mean, 0.87 mg/m^3; 95% confidence interval, 0.65—1.16). The concentrations in factory air between 1973 and 1980 ranged between 0.031 and 2.9 mg/m^3. Female spot welders had the highest concentrations of cadmium in blood (154.6 µg/L) and urine (78.8 µg/L).

Average airborne concentrations of *cadmium oxide* measured in a cadmium refining plant in Hunan Province, China, ranged from 0.004 to 0.187 mg/m^3 at most work sites. The average cadmium level in the blood of 65 workers at the plant in 1982 was 20.4 µg/L (range, 1.0—92.5) (Liu et al., 1985).

A cross-sectional study of lead and *cadmium* poisoning was carried out in Salvador, Bahia, Brazil, among 39 workers employed in repairing batteries from motor vehicles in 19 small establishments (Carvalho et al., 1985). Levels of cadmium were very high (geometric mean, 0.074 µmol/L; range, 0.004—0.247); those in 38 workers were greater than 0.009 µmol/L. High levels of cadmium in blood were associated with worker's age, amount of time spent repairing batteries, poor ventilation of the work area and work in small enterprises.

A retrospective cohort study was conducted in seven large cities of China that included information on 2982 workers exposed to *chromate* in seven chromate manufacturing plants (Wu, 1988). The few available data indicated that exposure to chromate during 1963—80 varied between 0.02 and 21.3 mg/m^3. Air chromate levels at some work sites were reported to have been much higher at times.

The ore mined by the Yunnan Tin Corporation in the Gejiu area of Yunnan Province, China, is a complex mixture of minerals; the precise mineral content varies by mine, the area within the mine and the distance from the surface. The predominant component of the ore is iron oxides, but air measurements after 1977 showed median concentrations of < 0.05 µg/m^3 *cadmium*, 0.075 µg/m^3 *nickel* and < 0.55 µg/m^3 *chromium* (Taylor et al., 1989).

Ionizing radiation

Occupational exposures to radiation were measured among workers in nuclear reactor plants in Taiwan Province, China, for the period 1962—83 (Weng & Chen, 1985). The total number of workers monitored ranged from 251 in 1962 to over 4000 in the 1980s. The highest collective dose equivalent was noted in 1981 and was estimated to be 5353 person-Sv; the average measurable dose equivalent per worker was 0.0025 Sv, and the maximal individual dose equivalent was 0.1 Sv.

Monitoring of radon underground in the Gejiu tin mine in Yunnan, China started in 1972 (Sun, 1988). The highest average value found was 2.9 × 10 000 Bq/m^3 (780 pCi/L); the estimated concentration of radon daughters was 5.4 WL, and the unattached fraction of radon daughters was 0.018—0.034, depending on the existing dust concentration. It was suggested that the value obtained in 1972 (5 WL) represents typical exposure levels for Gejiu miners before 1950.

Exposure to radon among Chinese tin miners was evaluated by estimating work-months of exposure based on job histories and industrial hygiene data and by measuring ^{210}Pb activity in the skull. Levels ranged from minimal to above 107.4 Bq (Laurer *et al.*, 1993).

Exposure to ionizing radiation was reported among workers in Koko, Nigeria, working in a waste dump containing radioactive and toxic wastes, among whom radiation-induced haematological injury was reported. It was estimated that exposure was lower than 0.31 Ci/kg (Ogunranti, 1989).

Concluding remarks

Many reports and published manuscripts describe the presence of occupational exposures to carcinogens but do not provide levels of exposure. These exposures include many recognized carcinogens and all the industrial chemicals, occupations and industrial processes classified by IARC working groups into Groups 1 and 2A.

In those industries in developing countries in which exposure has been measured, the levels (Tables 4–9) are relatively high and generally exceed the regulatory levels in industrialized countries. It therefore seems reasonable to assume that similar patterns apply to those industries and exposures for which reliable measurements have not been reported. It is of particular concern that there are relatively high levels of exposure to chemicals, such as benzidine-based dyes, that have been banned in industrialized countries.

Average individual levels of exposure to asbestos and benzene appear to have decreased over time in developing countries (see Figures 3 and 4), as in industrialized countries. Thus, the absolute differences in average levels of exposure between developing and industrialized countries have decreased; however, the relative differences (i.e. the ratio of average exposure levels in developing and industrialized countries) have often increased. Furthermore, the numbers of workers in many of these industries are increasing rapidly as a result of the transfer of hazardous industries from industrialized to developing countries (see Chapter 2). Thus, the total exposure of the work-force in developing countries to carcinogens is currently greater than at any time in the past.

References

Aksoy, M., Erdem, S. & Dinçol, G. (1974) Leukemia in shoeworkers exposed chronically to benzene. *Blood*, **44**, 837–841

Aksoy, M., Ozeris, S., Sabuncu, H., Inanici, Y. & Yanardag, R. (1987) Exposure to benzene in Turkey between 1983 and 1985: a haematological study on 231 workers. *Br. J. Ind. Med.*, **44**, 785–787

Amasa, S.K. (1975) Arsenic pollution at Obuasi goldmine, town, and surrounding countryside. *Environ. Health Perspectives*, **12**, 131–135

Arroyave, M.E. (1993) Pulmonary obstructive disease in a population using paraquat in Colombia. In: Forget, G., Goodman, T. & de Villiers, A., eds, *Impact of Pesticide Use on Health in Developing Countries*, Ottawa, International Development Research Center, pp. 76–84

Baker, E.L., Jr, Zack, M., Miles, J.W., Alderman, L., Warren, M., Dobbin, R.D., Miller, S. & Teeters, W.R. (1978) Epidemic malathion poisoning in Pakistan malaria workers. *Lancet*, **i**, 31–34

Baloyi, R. (1989) *Exposure to Asbestos among Chrysotile Miners, Millers and Mine Residents and Asbestosis in Zimbabwe*, Helsinki, Institute of Occupational Health

Berman, D.M. (1986) Asbestos and health in the third world: the case of Brazil. *Int. J. Health Serv.*, **16**, 253–263

Bi, W., Hayes, R.B., Feng, P., Qi, Y., You, X., Zhen, J., Zhang, M., Qu, B., Fu, Z., Chen, M., Co Chien, H.T. & Blot, W.J. (1992) Mortality and incidence of bladder cancer in benzidine-exposed workers in China. *Am. J. Ind. Med.*, **21**, 481–489

Carvalho, F.M., Silvany-Neto, A.M., Lima, M.E.C., Tavares, T.M. & Alt, F. (1985) Lead and cadmium poisoning among workers in small establishments for repairing batteries in Salvador, Brazil. *Rev. Saude Publ. S. Paulo*, **19**, 411–420 (in Portuguese)

Chen, O.Y., Tan, K.T., Kwok, S.F. & Chio, L.F. (1982) Study on workers exposed to cadmium in alkaline storage battery manufacturing and PVC compounding. *Ann. Acad. Med.*, **11**, 122–130

Chen, J., McLaughlin, J.K., Zhang, J.-Y., Stone, B.J., Luo, J., Chen, R.-A., Dosemeci, M., Rexing, S.H., Wu, Z., Hearl, F.J., McCawley, M.A. & Blot, W.J. (1992) Mortality among dust-exposed Chinese mine and pottery workers. *J. Occup. Med.*, **34**, 311–316

Cheng, W.-N. & Kong, J. (1992) A retrospective mortality cohort study of chrysotile asbestos products workers in Tianjin 1972–1987. *Environ. Res.*, **59**, 271–278

Cheng, V.K.I. & O'Kelly, F.J. (1986) Asbestos exposure in the motor vehicle repair and servicing industry in Hong Kong. *J. Soc. Occup. Med.*, **36**, 104–106

Condarco Aguilar, C., Medina, H., Chinchilla, J., Veneros, N., Aguilar, M. & Carranza, F. (1993) Pesticide poisoning among agricultural workers in Bolivia. In: Forget, G., Goodman, T. & de Villiers, A., eds, *Impact of Pesticide Use on Health in Developing Countries*, Ottawa, International Development Research Centre, pp. 76–84

Copplestone, J.F., Fakhri, Z.I., Miles, J.W., Mitchell, C.A., Osman, Y. & Wolfe, H.R. (1976) Exposure to pesticides in agriculture: a survey of spraymen using dimethoate in the Sudan. *Bull. World Health Organ.*, **54**, 217–223

Cullen, M.R. & Baloyi, R.S. (1991) Chrysotile asbestos and health in Zimbabwe: I. Analysis of miners and millers compensated for asbestos-related diseases since independence (1980). *Am. J. Ind. Med.*, **19**, 161–169

Cullen, M.R., Lopez-Carrillo, L., Alli, B., Pace, P.E., Shalat, S.L. & Baloyi, R.S. (1991) Chrysotile asbestos and health in Zimbabwe: II. Health status survey of active miners and millers. *Am. J. Ind. Med.*, **19**, 171–182

Das, M., Bhargava, S.K., Kumar, A., Khan, A., Bharti, R.S., Pangtey, B.S., Rao, G.S. & Pandya, K.P. (1991) An investigation of environmental impact on health of workers at retail petrol pumps. *Ann. Occup. Hyg.*, **35**, 347–352

Dewan, A., Jani, J.P., Patel, J.S., Gandhi, D.N., Variya, M.R. & Ghodasara, N.B. (1988) Benzidine and its acetylated metabolites in the urine of workers exposed to Direct Black 38. *Arch. Environ. Health*, **43**, 269–272

Dover, M.J. (1985) *A Better Mousetrap: Improving Pest Management for Agriculture*, Washington DC, World Resources Institute

Edwards, C.A. (1986) Agrochemicals as environmental pollutants. In: Hofsten, B.V. & Ekstrom, G., eds, *Control of Pesticide Applications and Residues in Food — A Guide and Directory 1986*, Uppsala, Swedish Science Press

Faria, M.M. (1987) Haematological values in workers exposed to benzene. *Boletim*, **9**, 100–105 (in Portuguese)

de Fernicola, N.G.G., Wakamatsu, C.T., Mendes, R. & Moraes, E.deC.F. (1976) Urinary output of phenol in workmen exposed to benzene in the shoe industry. *Rev. Saude Publ.*, **10**, 327–333 (in Portuguese)

Forget, G. (1991) Pesticides and the Third World. *J. Toxicol. Environ. Health*, **32**, 11–31

Foundation for Advancements in Science and Education (1993) Exporting banned and hazardous pesticides, 1991 statistics. The second export survey by the FASE pesticide project. *FASE Rep.*, **11** (Suppl.), S1–S8

Gibbs, G.W. & du Toit, R.S.J. (1973) Environmental data in mining. In: Bogovski, P., Gilson, J.C., Timbrell, V. & Wagner, J.C., eds, *Biological Effects of Asbestos* (IARC Scientific Publications No. 8), Lyon, IARC, pp. 138–144

Goldsmith, J.R. (1985) Occupational health in Chinese metallurgical industries: report based on a visit. *Am. J. Ind. Med.*, **7**, 353–357

Harper, M. & Possel Miranda, G. (1990) Management of health risks in the arsenic production industry: modern production in Chile in the context of past experience in Britain. *Ann. Occup. Hyg.*, **34**, 471–482

He, F., Sun, J., Han, K., Wu, Y., Tao, P., Wang, S. & Lin, L. (1988) Effects of pyrethroid insecticides on subjects engaged in packaging pyrethroids. *Br. J. Ind. Med.*, **45**, 548–551

Hein, R., Aung, B.U.T., Lwin, O. & Zaidi, S.H. (1989) Assessment of occupational benzene exposure in petrol filling stations at Rangoon. *Ann. Occup. Hyg.*, **33**, 133–136

Ho, S.F., Lee, H.P. & Phoon, W.H. (1987) Malignant mesothelioma in Singapore. *Br. J. Ind. Med.*, **44**, 788–789

Howard, J.K., Sabapathy, N.N. & Whitehead, P.A. (1981) A study of the health of Malaysian plantation workers with particular reference to paraquat spraymen. *Br. J. Ind. Med.*, **38**, 110–116

Huang, J.Q. (1990) A study on the dose–response relationship between asbestos exposure level and asbestosis among workers in a Chinese chrysotile product factory. *Biomed. Environ. Sci.*, **3**, 90–98

Huang, W.-Y. & Zhang, S.-Z. (1988) A survey on the occupational health situations in rural industries. In: Xue, S.-Z. & Liang, Y.-X., eds, *Occupational Health in Industrialization and Modernization* (Bulletin of WHO Collaborating Centre for Occupational Health, Shanghai, Vol. 2), Shanghai, Shanghai Medical University Press, pp. 137–142

IARC (1991) *IARC Monographs on the Evaluation of Carcinogenic Risks to Humans*, Vol. 53, *Occupational Exposures in Insecticide Application, and Some Pesticides*, Lyon

Indian National Institute of Occupational Health (1989–90) *Annual Report*, Ahmedabad

Ives, J.H. (1986) The health effects of the transfer of technology to the developing world: report and case studies. In: Ives, J.H., ed., *The Export of Hazard: Transnational Corporations and Environmental Control Issues*, London, Routledge & Kegan Paul, pp. 172–191

Jeyaratnam, J. (1985a) Health problems of pesticide usage in the Third World. *Br. J. Ind. Med.*, **42**, 505–506

Jeyaratnam, J. (1985b) 1984 and occupational health in developing countries. *Scand. J. Work Environ. Health*, **11**, 229–234

Jeyaratnam, J. (1992) Acute pesticide poisoning and developing countries. In: Jeyaratnam, J., ed., *Occupational Health in Developing Countries*, Oxford, Oxford University Press, pp. 255–264

Johannig, E., Selikoff, I.J. & Goldberg, M. (1991) *Asbestos Health Hazard Evaluation in South Korea. Asbestos Textile Manufacturing*, New York, Mount Sinai Medical Center

Kato, M., Rocha, M.L.R., Carbalho, A.B., Chaves, M.E.C., Raña, M.C.M. & Oliveira, F.C. (1993) Occupational exposure to neurotoxicants: prelimary survey in five industries of the Camaçari Petrochemical Complex in Brazil. *Environ. Res.*, **61**, 133–139

Lam, W.K., Kung, T.M., Ma, P.L., So, S.Y. & Mok, C.K. (1983) First report of asbestos-related diseases in Hong Kong. *Trop. Geogr. Med.*, **35**, 225–229

Laurer, G.R., Gang, Q.T., Lubin, J.H., Huna-Yao, L., Kan, C.S., Xiang, Y.S., Jian, C.Z., Yi, H., De, G.W. & Blot, W.J. (1993) Skeletal ^{210}Pb levels and lung cancer among radon-exposed tin miners in southern China. *Health Phys.*, **64**, 253–259

Levy, B.S. & Seplow, A. (1992) Asbestos-related hazards in developing countries. *Environ. Res.*, **59**, 167–174

Liu, Y.-Z., Huang, J.-X., Luo, C.-M., Xu, B.-H. & Zhang, C.-J. (1985) Effects of cadmium on cadmium smelter workers. *Scand. J. Work Environ. Health*, **11** (Suppl. 4), 29–32

Liu, X.-Z., Lo, S.-C., Wang, M.-Z., Yu, M.-H. & Liu, P.-L. (1988) An investigation on the mesothelioma occurred in a rural area with heavy crocidolite contamination. In: Xue, S.-Z. & Liang, Y.-X., eds, *Occupational Health in Industrialization and Modernization* (Bulletin of WHO Collaborating Centre for Occupational Health, Shanghai, Vol. 2), Shanghai, Shanghai Medical University Press, pp. 148–149

Loevinsohn, M.E. (1987) Insecticide use and increased mortality in rural central Luzon, Philippines. *Lancet*, **i**, 1359–1362

Lou, J. & Zhou, C. (1989) The prevention of silicosis and prediction of its future prevalence in China. *Am. J. Public Health*, **79**, 1613–1616

Lum, K.Y., Jusoh Mamat, M.D., Cheah, U.B., Castaneda, C.P., Rola, A.C. & Sinhasen, P. (1993) Pesticide research for public health and safety in Malaysia, the Philippes and Thailand. In: Forget, G., Goodman, T. & de Villiers, A., eds, *Impact of Pesticide Use on Health in Developing Countries*, Ottawa, International Development Research Centre, pp. 31–48

McDermott, M., Bevan, M.M., Elmes, P.C., Allardice, J.T. & Bradley, A.C. (1982) Lung function and radiographic change in chrysotile workers in Swaziland. *Br. J. Ind. Med.*, **39**, 338–343

McLaughlin, J.K., Chen, J.-Q., Dosemeci, M., Chen, R.-A., Rexing, S.H., Wu, Z., Hearl, F.J., McCawley, M.A. & Blot, W.J. (1992) A nested case–control study of lung cancer among silica exposed workers in China. *Br. J. Ind. Med.*, **49**, 167–171

Mohamed, I.Y. (1990) Asbestos–cement pneumoconiosis: first surgically confirmed case in Kuwait. *Am. J. Ind. Med.*, **17**, 241–245

Mukherjee, A.K., Rajmohan, H.R., Dave, S.K., Rajan, B.K., Kakde, Y. & Raghavendra Rao, S. (1992) An environmental survey in chrysotile asbestos milling processes in India. *Am. J. Ind. Med.*, **22**, 543–551

Mwanthi, M.A. & Kimani, V.N. (1993) Agrochemicals: a potential health hazard among Kenya's small-scale farmers. In: Forget, G., Goodman, T. & de Villiers, A., eds, *Impact of Pesticide Use on Health in Developing Countries,* Ottawa, International Development Research Centre, pp. 106–113

Noweir, M.H. (1986) Occupational health in developing countries with special reference to Egypt. *Am. J. Ind. Med.*, **9**, 125–141

Ogaram, D. (1990) Potential hazards in Uganda (silicosis, asbestosis, etc.). *East Afr. Newslett.*, **1**, 10–11

Ogunranti, J.O. (1989) Haematological indices in Nigerians exposed to radioactive waste. *Lancet*, **ii**, 667–668

Oleru, U.G. (1980) Pulmonary function of control and industrially exposed Nigerians in asbestos, textile, and toluene diisocyanate-foam factories. *Environ. Res.*, **23**, 137–148

Oleru, U.G. & Onyekwere, C. (1992) Exposures to polyvinyl chloride, methyl ketone and other chemicals. *Int. Arch. Environ. Health*, **63**, 503–507

Prinsen, G.H. & Van Sittert, N.J. (1980) Exposure and medical monitoring study of a new synthetic pyrethroid after one season of spraying on cotton in Ivory Coast. In: Tordoir, W.F. & van Heemstra-Lequin, E.A.H., eds, *Field Worker Exposure During Pesticide Application* (Studies in Environmental Science No. 7), Amsterdam, Elsevier, pp. 105–120

Qiao, Y.-L., Taylor, P.R., Yao, S.-X., Schatzkin, A., Mao, B.-L., Lubin, J., Rao, J.-Y., McAdams, M., Xuan, X.-Z. & Li, J.-Y. (1989) Relation of radon exposure and tobacco use to lung cancer among tin miners in Yunnan Province, China. *Am. J. Ind. Med.*, **16**, 511–521

Rees, D. & Kielkowski, D. (1991) Dust and pneumoconiosis in the South African ceramic industry. *S. Afr. J. Sci.*, **87**, 493–495

Romo-Kroger, C.M., Morales, R., Llona, F., Auriol, P. & Wolleter, G.E. (1989) Risks of airborne particulate exposure in a copper mine in Chile. *Ind. Health*, **27**, 95–99

Sakari, W.D.O. (1990) Occupational lung disorders due to mineral dusts in Kenya. *East Afr. Newslett.*, **1**, 6–7

Sansur, R.M., Kuttab, S. & Abu-Al-Haj, S. (1993) Extent of exposure of farm workers to organophosphate pesticides in the Jordan Valley. In: Forget, G., Goodman, T. & de Villiers, A., eds, *Impact of Pesticide Use on Health in Developing Countries*, Ottawa, International Development Research Centre, pp. 131–140

Solomons, K. (1984) Malignant mesothelioma — clinical and epidemiological features. A report of 80 cases. *S. Afr. Med. J.*, **66**, 407–412

Sun, S. (1988) Etiology of lung cancer at the Gejiu tin mine, China. In: Miller, R.W., Watanabe, S., Fraumeni, J.F., Jr, Sugimura, T., Takayama, S. & Sugano, H., eds, *Unusual Occurrences as Clues to Cancer Etiology*, Tokyo, Japan Scientific Society Press, pp. 103–115

Taylor, P.R., Qiao, Y.-L., Schatzkin, A., Yao, S.-X., Lubin, J., Bao, B.-L., Rao, J.-Y., McAdams, M., Xuan, X.-Z. & Li, J.-Y. (1989) Relation of arsenic exposure to lung cancer among tin miners in Yunnan Province, China. *Br. J. Ind. Med.*, **46**, 881–886

United Nations (1971) *UN Statistical Yearbook*, New York

United Nations (1975) *UN Statistical Yearbook*, New York

United Nations (1983) *UN Statistical Yearbook*, New York

United Nations (1987) *UN Statistical Yearbook*, New York

Venkataraman, N. (1982) Socio-economic impact of asbestos use (cost–benefit analysis) with special reference to developing countries. In: *Proceedings of the World Symposium on Asbestos, 25–27 May 1982, Montreal*, Montreal, Canadian Asbestos Information Centre, pp. 224–230

Weng, P.-S. & Chen, T.-C. (1985) Occupational radiation exposures in Taiwan, 1962–1983. *Health Phys.*, **49**, 411–418

White, N.W., Chetty, R. & Bateman, E.D. (1991) Silicosis among gemstone workers in South Africa: tiger's eye pneumoconiosis. *Am. J. Ind. Med.*, **19**, 205–213

WHO (1973) *Safe Use of Pesticides. Twentieth Report of the WHO Expert Committee on Insecticides* (WHO Technical Report Series No. 513), Geneva

World Resources Institute (1986) *World Resources: A Report by the World Resources Institute and the International Institute for Environment and Development 1986*, New York, Basic Books

Wu, W. (1988) Occupational cancer epidemiology in the People's Republic of China. *J. Occup. Med.*, **30**, 968–974

Yang, M.-D., Wang, J.-D., Wang, Y.-L., Guo, P.-S., Yao, Z.-Q., Lu, P.-L., Gu, X.-Y., Dong, Y.-L., Lu, M.-X., Zhu, P., Tan, S.-G., Liu, Q.-P., Jiang, M.-C., Chen, Z.-Q., Fang, S.-Q., Ren, S.-Y., Shen, D., Qiao, T.-Y., Huang, F.-S. & Jiang, Z.-D. (1985) Changes in health conditions in the Huainan coal mine in the past three decades. *Scand. J. Work Environ. Health*, **11** (Suppl. 4), 64–67

Yin, S.-N., Li, Q., Liu, Y., Tian, F., Du, C. & Jin, C. (1987) Occupational exposure to benzene in China. *Br. J. Ind. Med.*, **44**, 192–195

Zhang, R.-W. & Jiang, X.-Z. (1988) A preliminary report on the analysis of malignant mortality among anatomists and their assistants. In: Xue, S.-Z. & Liang, Y.-X., eds, *Occupational Health in Industrialization and Modernization* (Bulletin of WHO Collaborating Centre for Occupational Health, Shanghai, Vol. 2), Shanghai, Shanghai Medical University Press, pp. 89–90

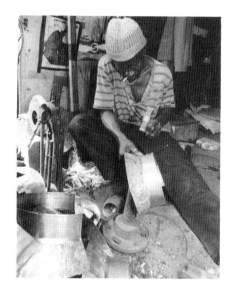

Exposures are especially difficult to control in small workshops where the work-force often includes young children.

Above: Scrap metal being converted into kitchen utensils.

Photo by J. Maillard, courtesy of International Labour Office

Below: Young Mexicans help in their family's copperware workshop.

Photo by D. Bregnard, courtesy of World Health Organization and International Labour Office

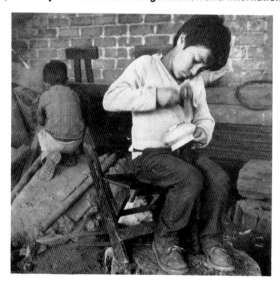

Chapter 6. Special Exposure Circumstances

This chapter comprises two reviews of information on special exposure circumstances that may be particularly hazardous owing either to the extent of exposure or to the susceptibility of the exposed population: the first section reviews information on exposures in small-scale industries, and the second examines the problem of child labour.

Small-scale industries (R. Loewenson)

Introduction

Small industries have been estimated to employ about one-half of the work-force in manufacturing and related industries in developing countries (Reverente, 1992). Generally, the smaller the industry is, the higher the rate of workplace injury and illness. Working conditions, hygiene and safety in these enterprises are often poor, and the workplaces are often characterized by old machinery, noise, unsafe buildings and other structures, employees with limited education, skill and training and employers with limited financial resources. Protective clothing, respirators, gloves, hearing protectors and safety glasses are seldom available. The companies tend to be scattered geographically and therefore inaccessible to inspection by labour groups or government health and safety enforcement agencies (LaDou, 1991). The number of workers employed in each unit is usually small, and their health status is often a direct reflection of the level of health in the population (Noweir, 1986).

Small-scale workplaces may be located in or near homes, and measures to protect not only workers but also nearby residents from hazardous exposures are often lacking. Workers in such businesses include large, vulnerable population groups such as children (see below), youths, women and the elderly, who generally earn less than the minimum wage and come from lower social strata. In general, such employees do not have ready access to health benefits and, like unemployed and workers in the informal sector, are not covered by health services. Such groups have been identified in Latin America as requiring urgent occupational health care (PAHO, 1990).

The majority of Africans work in small businesses, on small-holdings and in enterprises with fewer than five people. Employment statistics for the small-scale sector, also called the 'informal sector' in some countries, are often not available, given the frequently informal nature of employment contracts, use of family labour, including child labour, and the undefined boundary that often exists between informal-sector, small-scale employment and unemployment, with people moving more easily between these sectors than into the formal sector. Recent economic trends, including the introduction of structural adjustment programmes, appear to have increased the relative size of the small-scale sector, as larger enterprises in the formal sector have become more capital intensive and have shed labour through retrenchment and shifts to nonpermanent employment (Cornia *et al.*, 1987).

The major small-scale sector is agriculture, and the majority of African rural populations are engaged in farming on small holdings, often as a blend of commercial and subsistence crop production. Other forms of small-scale enterprise include mining and gold panning, craft work, small-scale industries, vending, trading and local services, including traditional health care and provision of services ranging from transport to hairdressing. The small-scale sector not only employs most of the poor in the population but is often the marketplace through which they procure the basic commodities for survival. Hence, many Africans are both producers and consumers within the sector. Because workers and farmers in Africa live next to many of the small-scale, informal-sector enterprises, there is a close link between working and living environments.

The health effects of production in the small-scale sector, and specifically the effects on cancer incidence, involve three elements: exposures in the work environment, exposures due to consumption of products from the small-scale sector and exposures due to contamination of the living environment by the work environment.

The following sections cover potential hazards in the small-scale sector, issues in the control of such hazards, including legal controls, and the provision of occupational health services. Finally, some key issues are identified in the prevention and management of occupational cancer in the small-scale sector in Africa. The African case is given as an example of problems that may be found in the small-scale sector of the economy in developing countries on other continents.

Occupational exposures

Workers in small enterprises face the range of hazards experienced in larger enterprises, physical (noise, heat, dust, electrical), chemical (pesticides, solvents, acids, resins), mechanical (cutting, grinding and other tools, vehicles), ergonomic (poor working platforms and positions) and biological (such as animal-borne disease and injury in farm work with animal draught power), as well as problems related to the organization of the work. Informal-sector workers often have poorer access to clean workplaces, toilets and adequate water.

Small-scale farmers are exposed to agrochemicals, owing particularly to increased pressure for fertilizer and pesticide use with shifts in crop production, use of hybrid seeds and the need to increase yields to match input costs. Small-scale farmers commonly apply chemicals manually using old, poorly maintained equipment. Thus, not only are exposures to chemicals increased, but ergonomic hazards are involved, owing to use of primitive handtools, hoes and ploughs, lifting heavy loads and sustained physical work.

The common factors that undermine workplace safety in these situations are:

-   low levels of capital, use of primitive tools and techniques and a tendency to in-novate or take shortcuts in production that, while necessary for economic survival, may pose serious hazards to the worker;

-   poor working conditions, poorly regulated by labour or health and safety laws and poorly monitored by unions, employers' organizations and the state, as workers such as those working for their 'families' are not always under formal contracts of employment. These problems are particularly acute in the categories of labour common in informal and small-scale enterprises, such as child, casual, family and female labour; the majority of smallholders and a large proportion of informal-sector workers are female, while many small rural and urban enterprises also employ children; and

-   poor access to information, lack of knowledge about hazards, their effects and controls and pressure to generate an income 'at whatever cost'.

Within this general framework, workers in small-scale enterprises are also exposed to carcinogens in a range of processes, which include: (i) agriculture, where pesticides are heavily used; for example, arsenic-based insecticides may be used, and agents such as DDT used in malarial control may be present at residual levels in the rural environment; (ii) the manufacture and use of asbestos-containing products, including roof sheeting, pipes and brake and clutch linings; (iii) processes involving benzidine and naphthylamine dyes; (iv) tyre-retread workshops, in which benzene and aromatic amines may be present; (v) leather and shoe manufacture, in which workers may be exposed to leather dust and benzene; and (vi) woodworking processes, where there is exposure to wood dust.

Indirect exposures may occur when larger-scale enterprises subcontract to small-scale businesses for the disposal of wastes that may include carcinogenic substances (e.g. asbestos waste), the laundering of work clothing that may be contaminated with chemical residues or the packaging and distribution of products containing carcinogens.

Consumption of products marketed in the small-scale sector may also pose problems. Pesticide residues on food products may result in exposure of nonoccupational groups, particularly in the case of organochlorine pesticides. Aflatoxins arising from fungal infection of food crops under humid conditions of production and storage have been associated with liver cancer (Tomatis *et al.*, 1990; Nyathi *et al.*, 1992; IARC, 1993). While screening for aflatoxins may be possible in the case of centralized marketing boards, it is less easy in small-scale vending operations.

Occupational use of carcinogenic agents may affect the general population when work environments are close to living environments, such as in agriculture. For example, high levels of organochlorine compounds have been found in breast milk in certain developing countries (Johnson, 1986). While waste from large-scale, formal-sector processes is a more substantial risk for communities adjacent to mining, processing and agricultural enterprises, unregulated environmental contamination from small-scale production also poses a potential hazard.

Controlling occupational hazards

Detection and control of occupational exposures depends on a system of monitoring and management at the level of the workplace and at the national level. In Africa, factory inspectorate systems have inadequate staff and resources to implement laws relating to the work environment, which are themselves often neither specific nor comprehensive. Countries such as Kenya, Mauritius, the Seychelles and Zimbabwe are now establishing laws and practices for workplace safety committees in order to localize monitoring and to promote legislative obligations for the dissemination of hazard information to manufacturers and employers.

A small-scale enterprise may not fulfil the definition of a 'factory' in the law governing inspections (such as in Zimbabwe) or may not *de facto* be monitored owing to shortages of inspectors, time and transport (Sitas *et al.*, 1988). A small-scale enterprise may have too few workers to be required legally to have a safety committee (such as in Namibia and Mauritius). Workers and employers in such enterprises are less well organized and thus less well informed of their rights to health and safety, of advances in work environment practices and of workplace hazards (ILO/WHO, 1990), greatly inhibiting effective monitoring of exposures. As shown in the previous chapter, few good assessments are therefore available of the pattern of occupational exposures and particularly of the chemicals used in this sector, and we are forced to rely on anecdotal evidence and cross-sectional studies. Those studies that have been carried out, e.g. that of Sakari (1991) in small-scale lead industries in Kenya, indicate high levels of exposure and poor working conditions.

Occupational health services

Detection of the health effects of occupational exposures depends on the accessibility of health services in general and particularly of screening for occupational illness, which are generally still underdeveloped in African countries. Workers in the small-scale sector often represent the poorer section of the population, who do not have workplace-based health care or health insurance and are limited in the use of health care by geographical and cost factors. They may rely more heavily on self-help, traditional health sectors and primary health care services, where knowledge of occupational health may be poor. Diagnosis of cancer, especially of internal organs, demands skills and supporting equipment that may be absent in the primary care facilities used by workers in small enterprises.

Since the labour force in this sector is relatively young, at risk for various communicable diseases and scattered, cancers may be preceded by other causes of death, or increased incidences in particular occupational groups may not be recognized. The AIDS epidemic not only contributes to lowering immunity and thus increasing the risk for ill health in African societies but may also complicate the detection of other disease processes.

Few workers in the small-scale sector are covered by workers' compensation. Even when laws provide that all workers under contract be covered by workers' compensation, the often undefined nature of employment contracts in small businesses and the lack of organization in and administrative control over the sector means that most workplaces are not covered. Hence, there is little legal impetus to monitor illness and injury in this sector on a routine basis, and, as with the monitoring of exposures, monitoring of the health impact of exposures is an ad-hoc, largely unregulated process.

Monitoring and managing occupational hazards and occupational cancer in small-scale enterprises

The above brief, somewhat qualitative discussion indicates certain basic issues that must be addressed if we are to monitor and manage more effectively occupational hazards in the small-scale sector, their health impact in general and, more specifically, their impact on occupational cancer:

Obtain a better data base: Most of the information on occupational health in the small-scale sector is qualitative; there is little systematic monitoring, and few surveys have been conducted. Given the large volume of employment in this sector, a better data base is needed on exposures and practices, their impact on health and potential resources available.

Organizational and administrative issues: Both workers and employers in the small-scale sector are highly disaggregated and badly organized in comparison with the formal sector, both internally and in relation to the state. Occupational health laws cover the sector inadequately or are poorly enforced; in order to create employment under structural adjustment programmes, there has been an even greater deregulation, which further weakens legal control in the sector. It is therefore difficult to establish traditional systems of promotion, dissemination of information, inspection and monitoring in small enterprises, and alternative approaches to occupational health development are needed.

The disaggregation of the sector must be overcome and collective systems of management be developed. For example, the provision by local authorities of appropriate shelters and work stations at agreed sites with proper toilet, water, electrical, ventilation, telephone and other facilities could provide a framework for information and support services on equipment, chemicals and safe work practices and easy access to the necessary spare parts and protective equipment. Such serviced work areas would also allow easier monitoring of environmental waste.

Reduce exposures: Many small-scale producers have shown their capacity to innovate work processes, sometimes providing solutions to occupational health problems. Kogi *et al.* (1989) compiled and documented 100 examples of 'low-cost ways of improving working conditions' in Asia, and similar work is in progress in East Africa. While this capacity should be tapped, it is not realistic to rely totally on the initiative and capacity of small-scale producers and employers to solve problems in the work environment. If they do not have the money, skills, mobility or time to resolve hazards associated with the use of equipment, the responsibility shifts to the manufacturers who furnish the sector. The inputs to small-scale producers should incorporate, as far as possible, basic safety features in design, low cost, use of local materials, easy maintenance and affordable, widely distributed spare parts. Labelling and safety instructions should be adequate and be written in local languages. Given the narrow profit margins, it is important to demonstrate that improving work environments through such methods improves output, in relation to both carcinogens and other occupational health risks.

A comprehensive approach: Occupational cancers cannot be singled out as an issue in the small-scale sector, given the general problems of public and occupational health that exist therein. Rather, the issue of occupational cancer should be part of general improvements in the work environment and public health. Because of the scattered nature of the sector and the mobile, informal and insecure nature of its labour force, occupational health initiatives in the workplace should probably be complemented by or located within more comprehensive, community-based health activities. The integration of occupational health and public health services in the small-scale sector raises the question of whether and how to link screening and management of occupational cancers in such enterprises with strategies for the prevention and control of more common public health-related cancers, such as cervical and liver cancer.

Dealing with these issues is not easy; however, until we address the occupational health needs in the small-scale sector, there can be no national occupational health strategies in African countries. It is a uniquely national challenge that we cannot afford to ignore.

Child labour in relation to occupational cancer (V. Forastieri and E. Matos)

Introduction

The origins of occupational medicine in the occidental part of the world can be traced to the first attempts to eliminate the worst abuses of child labour (Richter & Jacobs, 1991). Strategies for the prevention of work-related accidents and diseases are largely based on labour legislation and public health laws. Most standards for the minimum age of employment stem from knowledge about the health and development of children. The first clear-cut evidence of occupational cancer involved child labour (Checkoway *et al.*, 1989): Pott (1775) identified soot as the cause of scrotal cancer in London chimneysweeps and graphically described the abysmal working conditions, which involved children climbing up narrow chimneys that were still hot. Pott was greatly moved by the plight of his patients (quoted by Waldron, 1983):

> The fate of these people seems singularly hard; in their early infancy they are most frequently treated with great brutality, and almost starved with cold and hunger; they are thrust up narrow and sometimes hot chimneys, where they are buried, burned and almost suffocated; and when they get to puberty, become liable to a most noisome, painful and fatal disease.

Despite this evidence, reports of fires in chimneys were used to delay legislation on child labour in this industry until 1840 (Waldron, 1983). An experimental model of soot carcinogenesis was first demonstrated in the 1920s (Passey, 1922), 150 years after the original epidemiological observation (Decouflé, 1982).

Magnitude of the problem

Although child labour is now less common in many developed countries, it continues to be a source of concern; for example, more than 4 million children were employed in the USA in 1988 (Pollack *et al.*, 1990). Child labour appears to be more common in developing countries, which typically have young populations large percentages of which are below the age of 15. Child labour is rooted in poverty and is concentrated among people who live in conditions of absolute poverty, who have high mortality and morbidity rates, low life expectancy and poor access to health services. Estimates of the magnitude of the problem of child labour vary widely, owing to the use of different data sources and different definitions of 'child labour' and of 'economically active'. For example, ILO (1983) estimated that about 50 million children (under the age of 15) were 'economically active' at the beginning of the 1980s but commented that the figure could be as high as 75 or 100 million; other estimates are as high as 200 million (Pollack *et al.*, 1990). In 1983, ILO estimated that virtually all 'economically active' children (98%) lived in developing countries; in some countries, children constitute 15–25% of the total work-force (Pollack *et al.*, 1990).

Table 1 presents data from Richter and Jacobs (1991) based on provisional figures from the ILO for the early 1980s, which were obtained from censuses, official estimates and samples of the labour force. The highest frequency of child labour was found in Asia, particularly in India, Bangladesh, Pakistan and Indonesia. In non-Asian countries, child labour was commonest in Brazil, Ethiopia, Turkey, Mexico and Egypt. The figures are likely to be underestimates, because they are derived from official statistics that may be incomplete and often omit activities in the informal section, in which most children are engaged. For example, Tambellini (1986) estimated that children aged 10–14 constitute about 20% of the economically active population in Brazil, whereas the ILO estimate was around 14%. Conversely, El Batawi (1986) made estimates of only 20% in Bangladesh but as high as 38% in India, 32% in Mali, 30% in the United Republic of Tanzania, 25% in Thailand and 25% in Turkey.

Child labour is generally concentrated in agriculture, the services sector, small enterprises, family trades and the informal sector. Several studies have shown that thousands of children work in hazardous industries, such as glass manufacture, construction, mining and quarrying. Few data are available, however, on the incidence and prevalence of work-related injuries and diseases among children in developing countries. Most of the studies do not provide specific information on levels of exposure to chemicals, dust, heavy metals, solvents and pesticides, nor on the health effects of these exposures (Richter & Jacobs, 1991). Exposure to carcinogens is likely to occur, however, in jobs that are usually assigned to children, such as cleaning with solvents, application of wood impregnation products, small painting jobs (priming coats), handling of adhesives, handling of flags to guide pesticide-spray aeroplanes and mixing, loading and applying pesticides. Protective equipment is seldom used. The main industries and occupations that are known to carry a carcinogenic risk and in which children are involved in developing countries include: agriculture, mining and quarrying, construction, textile manufacture, carpet weaving, leather production, wood processing, ceramics, glass, brick-making, slate-making, painting, metalwork, toy making (with exposure to plastics, dyes and paints), precious stones and gems production (with exposures to chromic oxide and silica), auto repair and petrol distribution (see Tables 6 and 7 in Chapter 4 for details of specific occupations, type of cancers and reported causative and suspected agents).

Little information is available on the magnitude of the international health problem of children working in hazardous industries, owing mainly to the relative inaccessibility of the population at risk, which is concentrated mainly in the informal

Table 1. Percentage of children economically active in some countries, 1980–84

Country	Year	Age range	No. of children	Percentage economically active	Source	Remarks
Argentina	1983	10–14	198 034	8.1	Official estimate	
Bangladesh	1981	10–14	6 047 256	52.0	Census	Provisional
Botswana	1981	10–14	12 947	10.8	Census	
Brazil	1980	10–14	1 922 218	14.2	Census	1% sample only
Cameroon	1982	0–14	215 500	5.7	Official estimate	
Colombia	1980	0–14	92 435	1.0	Household survey	
Ecuador	1982	12–14	64 957	6.3	Census	Sample only (size unspecified)
Egypt	1980	12–14	1 102 300	6.5	Labour force sample survey	
El Salvador	1980	10–14	85 727	13.6	Household survey	
Ethiopia	1980	10–14	1 599 200	42.1	Official estimate	Figures rounded to nearest 100
Greece	1982	10–14	9 800	1.3	Labour force sample survey	
Guatemala	1981	10–14	78 878	10.4	Census	2.5% sample only
Haiti	1982	10–14	138 823	24.0	Census	
Honduras	1983	10–14	78 755	14.8	Official estimate	
Hungary	1980	10–14	3 185	0.5	Census	
India	1981	0–14	13 592 366	5.2	Census	5% sample
Indonesia	1980	10–14	1 958 156	11.1	Census	
Korea, Republic of	1983	14	25 000	0.5	Labour force sample survey	
Malaysia	1980	10–14	125 789	7.7	Census	
Mexico	1980	10–14	1 121 816	12.1	Census	Provisional
Nepal	1981	10–14	972 698	57.0	Census	
Pakistan	1981	10–14	2 143 904	20.4	Census	Provisional, some states excluded

Table 1 (contd)

Country	Year	Age range	No. of children	Percentage economically active	Source	Remarks
Panama	1980	10–14	9 572	4.2	Census	Some areas excluded
Paraguay	1982	10–14	45 140	11.8	Census	10% sample only
Peru	1981	10–14	124 231	5.7	Census	
Portugal	1982	10–14	85 00	9.3	Labour force sample survey	Provisional adjusted
Samoa	1981	10–14	355	1.5	Census	Provisional
Sao Tome and Principe	1981	10–14	265	2.2	Census	Provisional
Senegal	1983	10–14	382 000	50.1	Official estimate	Provisional
Seychelles	1981	10–14	75	1.0	Official estimate	Provisional
Singapore	1983	10–14	2 095	0.9	Labour force sample	Provisional
Sri Lanka	1981	0–14	85 749	1.7	Labour force sample survey	
Syrian Arab Republic	1983	10–14	41 163	2.9	Labour force sample survey	
Thailand	1980	0–14	1 024 200	4.9	Labour force sample survey	Some unpaid family workers excluded
Togo	1980	0–14	86 13	7.8	Official estimate	
Turkey	1980	14	1 346 819	7.8	Census	1% sample

From Richter & Jacobs (1991), taken from ILO (1983)

sector in many different types of occupation, and to the fact that child labour is seldom legally recognized. Action by public health officials and the authorities is therefore limited.

The abolition of child labour has been one of the fundamental objectives of ILO since its creation. Within the framework of an international project on the elimination of child labour, launched in 1992, ILO is gathering data from various countries on health risks for children in hazardous work. They have requested information on studies that have been conducted or are in progress, preventive and remedial measures that are in force, pilot programmes and national practices concerning the consequences of the work-related hazards and risks to which working children are exposed. The data being gathered include the number of working children under the age of 15, by age group, size and type of enterprise; the types of hazardous activity, occupation or industry in which children are engaged; the numbers of children estimated to be working in each occupation and industry; and the associated occupational diseases. Analysis of this information should provide more accurate data on the health consequences of child labour.

Regulation

In spite of the existence in many developing countries of laws and regulations pertinent to activities and occupations involving exposure to carcinogens, children are often not covered, as the legislation applies only to people under contract of employment. Children are often not employed legally. Examples of national laws and regulations related to the employment of children in activities that involve exposure to carcinogens are those of Zaire, the Sudan and Colombia, which prohibit the employment of children in work involving the use of lead paint; of Argentina, Chile and the United Republic of Tanzania, which prohibit employment of children under the age of 18 in underground mining; of India, where child labour legislation covers factories, plantations and workshops where certain types of industrial processes are carried out; and of the Philippines, where a comprehensive list of occupations, processes and industries considered to be hazardous for children has been established (ILO, 1991).

Health effects

Limited information is available on how occupational exposures affect children's health and development. Richter and Jacobs (1991) analysed cause-specific death rates of children in Egypt, Mexico and the Philippines, where there are high rates of child employment. They noted, however, that deaths are probably underreported in those countries and that the rubric 'accidents' does not distinguish between those of occupational origin and other accidents, probably including deaths from work injury in agriculture — a notoriously underreported outcome in developing countries. The higher cause-specific death rates for respiratory diseases among children and youths may be a partial consequence of exposures to toxic and hazardous dusts and fibres, mists, gases and fumes, combined with the fact that their overall health is compromised by malnutrition, endemic diseases, poor hygiene and smoking. The data necesary to determine the role of hazardous occupational exposures in the mortality of older children are not, however, available. The authors stated that the data give no indication of the number of deaths from pesticide poisoning in working children and youths.

Although virtually none of the studies have addressed directly the possible health effects in child labourers of exposure to occupational carcinogens, the results of studies in adults obviously create concern. Furthermore, several factors may make exposure to occupational carcinogens more hazardous to children than to adults. Children differ structurally and functionally from adults in their morphological, physiological, biochemical and metabolic characteristics, because they are growing and developing. Their responses to chemicals and other hazardous agents therefore differ from those of adults. The effects of exposure also differ according to age, nutritional status and the chemical (e.g. characteristics, metabolism, degree of maturation of target organ). A similar dose of a chemical is likely to accumulate to a greater proportion per unit body weight in a child than in a young person or adult. If exposure starts in childhood rather than in adulthood, total lifetime exposure will generally be longer. Chemicals that reach the body early in life may produce delayed effects. Since cumulative exposure is strongly associated with the risks presented by carcinogens, such as asbestos (Pearce, 1988) and hazardous chemicals, exposure during childhood may result in particularly increased risks at older ages. Even for a given level of cumulative lifetime exposure, exposures during childhood may be more hazardous than exposures later in life if the carcinogen acts at an early stage of the cancer process (Pearce *et al.*, 1986). Finally, very young children may be more vulnerable to the acute effects of some occupational exposures and may therefore be more susceptible to chronic effects, such as cancer; however, little evidence exists currently to assess this hypothesis, as no epidemiological observations on human infants have been reported in which the occurrence of cancer was associated exclusively with exposure to carcinogens. The few existing data come from studies in experimental animals.

References

Checkoway, H.A., Pearce, N.E. & Crawford-Brown, D.F. (1989) *Research Methods in Occupational Epidemiology*, New York, Oxford University Press

Cornia, G., Jolly, J. & Stewart, F. (1987) *Adjustment with a Human Face*, Oxford, Clarendon Press

Decouflé, P. (1982) Occupation. In: Schottenfeld, D. & Fraumeni, J.F., Jr, eds, *Cancer Epidemiology and Prevention*, Philadelphia, W.B. Saunders, pp. 318–335

El Batawi, M.A. (1986) The third Theodore F. Hatch symposium lecture. *Ann. Am. Conf. Gov. Ind. Hyg.*, **14**, 3–15

IARC (1993) *IARC Monographs on the Evaluation of Carcinogenic Risks to Humans*, Vol. 56, *Some Naturally Occurring Substances: Food Items and Constituents, Heterocyclic Aromatic Amines and Mycotoxins*, Lyon, pp. 245–395

ILO (1983) *Report of the Director-General in the 69th Session of the International Labour Conference*, Geneva

ILO (1991) *Conditions of Work Digest*, Vol. 10, *Child Labour: Law and Practice*, Geneva

ILO/WHO (1990) *Proceedings of the East African Regional Symposium on Regulations and Control in Occupational Health and Safety 1989* (East African Newsletter on Occupational Health), Helsinki, Institute of Occupational Health

Johnson, E. (1986) Occupational cancer in developing countries. In: *Proceedings of the ILO–Finnish Symposium on Occupational Health and Safety in East Africa, Tanzania, November 1986*, pp. 21–30

Kogi, K., Phhon, W. & Thurman, J. (1989) *Low Cost Ways of Improving Working Conditions: 100 Examples from Asia*, Geneva, ILO

LaDou, J. (1991) The challenge of international occupational health. *International Commission on Occupational Health Q. Newslett.*, **10**, 2 May, 1–10

Noweir, M.H. (1986) Occupational health in developing countries with special reference to Egypt. *Am. J. Ind. Med.*, **9**, 125–141

Nyathi, C., Dube, N. & Hasler, J. (1992) Mycotoxins. *Afr. Newslett. Occup. Health Saf.*, **2** (Suppl. 1), 49–55

PAHO (1990) *Health Conditions in the Americas*, Vol. 1 (PAHO Scientific Publication 524), Washington DC

Passey, R.D. (1922) Experimental soot cancer. *Br. Med. J.*, **ii**, 1112–1113

Pearce, N. (1988) Multistage modelling of lung cancer mortality in asbestos textile workers. *Int. J. Epidemiol.*, **17**, 747–752

Pearce, N.E., Checkoway, H.A. & Shy, C.M. (1986) Time-related factors as potential confounders and effect modifiers in studies based on an occupational cohort. *Scand. J. Work Environ. Health*, **12**, 97–107

Pollack, S.H., Landrigan, P.J. & Mallino, D.L. (1990) Child labour in 1990: prevalence and health hazards. *Ann. Rev. Public Health*, **19**, 359–375

Pott, P. (1775) *Chirurgical Observations*, London, Hawes, Clarke and Collins

Reverente, B.R. (1992) Occupational health services for small-scale industries. In: Jeyaratnam, J., ed., *Occupational Health in Developing Countries*, Oxford, Oxford University Press, pp. 62–88

Richter, E.D. & Jacobs, J. (1991) Work injuries and exposures in children and young adults: review and recommendations for action. *Am. J. Ind. Med.*, **19**, 747–769

Sakari, W. (1991) Blood levels of workers in small scale lead industries in Kenya. *East Afr. Newslett.*, **Suppl. 1**, 69–70

Sitas, F., Davies, J., Kieikowski, D. & Becklake, M. (1988) Occupational health services in South African manufacturing industries: a pilot survey. *Am. J. Ind. Med.*, **14**, 545–557

Tambellini, A.T. (1986) *Politica Nacional de Saude do Trabalhador: Analises e Perspectivas* [National Policy for Occupational Health: Analyses and Perspectives], Rio de Janeiro, FIOCRUZ

Tomatis, L., Aitio, A., Day, N.E., Heseltine, E., Kaldor, J., Miller, A.B., Parkin, D.M. & Riboli, E., eds (1990) *Cancer: Causes, Occurrence and Control* (IARC Scientific Publications No. 100), Lyon, IARC

Waldron, H.A. (1983) A brief history of scrotal cancer. *Br. J. Ind. Med.*, **40**, 390–401

Part III

Health Effects

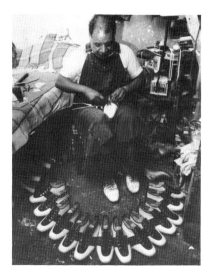

Exposure to known carcinogens is widespread in developing countries because of economic pressures and lack of awareness of hazards

Above: Shoe-makers are exposed to solvents, notably benzene

Photo: Courtesy of World Health Organization and International Labour Office

Below: The welding mask and gloves used by this young woman in the Philippines do not prevent inhalation of fumes containing metal oxides, ozone, oxides of nitrogen and organic compounds

Photo by J. Maillard, courtesy of International Labour Office

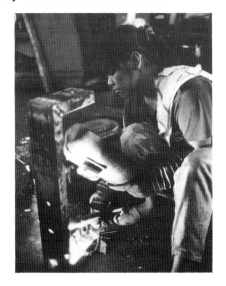

Chapter 7. Cancer

P. Boffetta, M. Kogevinas, N. Pearce and E. Matos

With few exceptions, little information is available on the occurrence of occupational cancer in developing countries. In this chapter, we review available information on asbestos, mining, silica, metalwork, coke production, benzene, vinyl chloride, rubber, chloromethyl methyl ether, textile manufacture, agriculture, ionizing radiation and other occupational exposures to carcinogens.

Exposures to asbestos

Relatively reliable information is available on cancer risks due to occupational exposure to asbestos and asbestos products in some developing countries. Studies on mortality from lung cancer in selected countries are summarized in Table 1.

Table 1. Mortality from lung cancer among asbestos-exposed workers in selected countries

Country	No. of workers	Exposure	No. of cases	SMR	Reference
South Africa	8 589	Crocidolite mining	86	1.64	Botha *et al.* (1986)
China	10 095	Asbestos product manufacture	129	6.33	Wu (1988)
China	6 198	Asbestos mining	Not reported	9.40	Wu (1988)
China	662 men	Asbestos textile manufacture	14	2.78	Cheng & Kong (1992)
	510 women		7	4.27	

SMR, standardized mortality ratio

South Africa

The first report on an association between exposure to asbestos and pleural mesothelioma came from South Africa, where a case of diffuse pleural mesothelioma with occasional clumps of asbestos bodies in the lung was discovered at autopsy in February 1956 (Wagner *et al.*, 1960). By the end of 1961, the authors had seen 67 cases from the Cape asbestos fields: 30 had had occupational exposure and a further eight had been exposed by working with asbestos outside the industry; 29 did not report occupational exposure to asbestos, but 22 were born on the Cape asbestos fields and nine had had industrial exposure to blue asbestos elsewhere in South Africa. For only two cases could neither a positive industrial nor environmental history be obtained. The youngest patient developed a mesothelioma at the age of 20: he had been exposed as a baby when his mother carried him on her back while she was cobbing asbestos fibres (for a historical review, see Wagner, 1991). Solomons (1984) reported the clinical and epidemiological features of 80 cases of malignant mesothelioma referred to the clinic at the South African National Centre for Occupational Health between January 1977 and June 1983. A positive history of exposure to asbestos was found in 89% of the cases. The types of asbestos involved were predominantly mixed, although Cape crocidolite was the sole type documented in 17 cases. The mean duration of exposure to asbestos was 13.6 years, and the mean lag period of time from first exposure to diagnosis was 34.3 years.

A survey was carried out on black miners at the Cape crocidolite mines in 1974. Of the 1185 employees or ex-employees recruited before July 1962, 215 had died before the survey and 215 could not be traced or data on them were incomplete; thus, 755 workers participated in the study. They were interviewed about their work history and received a clinical examination, a lung function test and an X-ray examination. About 70% of the study group had been exposed to asbestos for five years or less, but 96.3% of the workers had first been exposed more than 15 years previously. Four cases of mesothelioma of the pleura were found on initial examination, one more case was observed during the survey period and a further case was diagnosed after the survey was finished. In a second group of 947 ex-employees who were examined, 11 mesotheliomas of the pleura were found. Of a group of 53 women who had worked as hand-cobbers and who were examined at a hospital, 12 had pleural mesotheliomas (Talent *et al.*, 1980).

Standardized mortality ratios (SMRs) were calculated for selected causes of death among workers of white and mixed race in South African crocidolite mining districts between 1968 and 1980 (Botha *et al.*, 1986). Contiguous districts were used for comparison. High rates were observed of mesothelioma and of lung and stomach cancers. The SMRs were significantly elevated for both ethnic groups and both sexes, ranging from 7.86 to 10.30 for asbestosis and mesothelioma. The rates for lung cancer were significantly elevated for all groups except white females (SMRs, 1.31–1.45), and those for stomach cancer were significantly increased for mixed-race males and females (2.18 and 2.20, respectively). Mixed-race males also had statistically significant SMRs for malignant neoplasms of the lip, oral cavity and pharynx (2.72) and for cancer of the digestive organs (1.43). Only a small proportion of the population in the districts studied was employed in crocidolite mining, and the authors suggested that a major source of exposure to asbestos was environmental rather than occupational.

The incidence of mesothelioma was derived from a register of 1347 cases in South Africa for 1976–84 (Zwi *et al.*, 1989): 52% of the cases were in whites, 31% in blacks, 16% in mixed-race people and 1.5% in Asians; 73% of the cases were in males, 85% of whom had had prior exposure to asbestos, mainly occupational. The standardized incidence rates (SIRs) per million males per year were 32.9 (95% confidence interval [CI], 22.7−46.4) for whites, 24.8 (95% CI, 16.2−36.9) for coloureds and 7.6 (95% CI, 3.5−15.8) for blacks. The authors suggested that the differences in rates between ethnic groups reflected differences in detection, owing to differential access to health services.

Other countries

Two historical cohort studies, one on 10 095 workers manufacturing asbestos products and the other on 6198 asbestos miners, were conducted in China (Wu, 1988); information on exposure levels is given on p. 68. An excess risk for lung cancer was observed in both cohorts (SMR, 6.33; 90% CI, 4.74−8.30 for the first; SMR, 9.40; 90% CI, 6.10−14.16 for the second). The excess risk was found to be related to job, latency, extent of exposure and cigarette smoking.

More recently, lung cancer mortality was investigated in a cohort of 662 men and 510 women employed in asbestos textile, friction material and asbestos−cement manufacture in Tianjin, China (Cheng & Kong, 1992; see also p. 68). The cohort was followed for the period 1972−87. A significant excess for lung cancer mortality was found in both men (SMR, 2.78) and women (SMR, 4.3), and an increasing trend in SMR was observed with increasing intensity and duration of exposure. As in many studies of asbestos workers in industrialized countries, a synergistic effect (on an additive scale) on lung cancer mortality was observed between exposure to asbestos and cigarette smoking. The authors commented that the asbestos industry has developed in China since the 1950s and that mortality from lung cancer will increase as a consequence of exposure to both asbestos and cigarette smoke.

In Zimbabwe, four cases of asbestosis and two of mesothelioma were reported among railway workers (Mostert & Meintjes, 1979). All of the cases occurred in people who had not been exposed to high concentrations of asbestos dust, and in four of the six cases the only contact with any measurable quantity was with 3.2-mm asbestos string and 6.4-mm braid.

Among the approximately 300 men certified by the Zimbabwe Pneumoconiosis Bureau as having had occupational lung disease since 1984, 27 had findings consistent with one or more types of asbestos-associated disease (Cullen & Baloyi, 1991). Three died from malignancies, including one confirmed mesothelioma.

The first report of a malignant fibrous pleural mesothelioma in a Mexican worker was made in 1982 (Méndez Vargas *et al.*, 1982). The patient was exposed to chrysotile and crocidolite imported from Canada and South Africa.

Three cases of malignant mesothelioma and one case of asbestosis with small-cell carcinoma of the lung were identified at the University Department of Medicine, Queen Mary Hospital, Hong Kong, between 1976 and 1982 (Lam *et al.*, 1983). All had a history of occupational exposure to asbestos.

Nine cases of malignant mesothelioma were reported in Singapore over a 17-year period (Ho *et al.*, 1987; see p. 69). Detailed occupational histories were obtained for only two: both had worked in the same factory, where asbestos products were manufactured, had started work in the 1950s and had worked there for 15 and 17 years, respectively.

Mining

Selected cohort studies of miners are summarized in Table 2.

Table 2. Cohort studies of lung cancer among miners in developing countries

Country	No. of workers	Type of mining	Main exposures	No. of cases	SMR	Reference
South Africa	3 971	Gold	Silica, radon	39	1.6	Wyndham et al. (1986)
China	17 143	Tin	Radon, arsenic	Not reported[a]	10.4	Xuan et al. (1993)
China	Not reported	Haematite	Radon	29	3.7	Chen et al. (1990)

SMR, standardized mortality ratio

[a] Incidence

Coal mining

In a study of mortality among workers in the Huainan coal mine in eastern China (Yang et al., 1985; see p. 85), the unadjusted proportion of deaths from malignant tumours increased from 0.3% in 1953 to 5.6% in 1980, and that for cardiovascular diseases from 1.8 to 6.0%. The proportion of deaths from infectious diseases dropped from 17.3 to 12.1% during the same period.

Gold mining

In a study of 22 cases of carcinoma of the lung that occurred during 1948−56 in Africans in Gwanda, Zimbabwe (then Southern Rhodesia), Osburn (1957) noted that 13 patients had worked in mines, 12 in gold mines and one in an asbestos mine. Silica dust and arsenic were suggested as possibly relevant exposures.

The incidence of cancer among black South African gold miners was analysed for the period 1964−79 by area of residence (Bradshaw et al., 1982). In 2.9 million man-years of employment, 903 cancers were identified (about 360 per 100 000 per year): 45.6% were liver cancers, 19.8% oesophageal cancers, 11.2% respiratory cancers and 2.7% bladder cancers. The results for cancers at 11 other sites were presented by McGlashan et al. (1982).

A cohort of 3971 middle-aged, white South African gold miners was followed up for nine years, and SMRs were calculated in relation to the mortality of the entire white population of South Africa (Wyndham et al., 1986). The SMR for lung cancer was 1.61 (95% CI, 1.15−2.20). The smoking-adjusted relative risk (RR) estimated from a nested case−control study was 1.77 (0.94−3.31).

A case−control study performed on South African gold miners showed no association between exposure to silica dust and lung cancer or between lung cancer and silicosis (Hessel et al., 1986). Occupational exposure to silica dust was calculated by multiplying the number of shifts worked in a dusty atmosphere by a weighting factor proportional to the dust level in each occupation. The intensity of dust exposure was also calculated, weighted by the number of shifts at each level of intensity. A similar method of estimating exposure was used in a study of the mortality of 2209 white South African gold miners followed-up for 17 years (Hnizdo *et al.*, 1991). A dose—response relationship was found between death from lung cancer and exposure to silica dust: the highest RR was 2.9 (95% CI, 1.0—8.4) for more than 41 particle-years per 1000 (adjusted for smoking). An association was observed between mortality from lung cancer and silicosis of the hilar gland, but no association was seen with silicosis of the parenchyma or pleura.

Tin mining

The extremely high incidence of lung cancer among miners in Yunnan Province, China, was first noted in 1968. The highest rate for mortality from lung cancer among men, out of 2392 counties and cities in the country, was seen in Gejiu in a nationwide mortality survey conducted in 1973—75. Of the 1724 cases of lung cancer registered at the Yunnan Tin Corporation in the period 1954—86, 90% had a history of working underground. The crude annual incidence rate in 1983—85 among male miners aged 15 and over who had had underground exposure was 585/100 000 (Sun, 1988; Xuan *et al.*, 1991).

In an underground tin mine in Yunnan, in which exposure occurred to arsenic, radon decay products and ferric oxide (see pp. 85, 87, 90), 19% of all silicotics died from lung cancer (Goldsmith, 1985). In a case—control study on 107 prevalent cases of lung cancer among tin miners exposed to radon decay products in Yunnan (Qiao *et al.*, 1989; see pp. 90—91), people in the highest quartile of exposure had an odds ratio of 9.5 (95% CI, 2.7—33.1) when compared with people with no exposure to radon and after controlling for exposure to arsenic, age, year when starting work and tobacco use. The risk increased with duration of exposure. The same authors (Taylor *et al.*, 1989) examined exposure of these cases to arsenic (see p. 87). Subjects in the highest quartile of cumulative arsenic exposure had an RR of 22.6 when compared with subjects with no exposure, after adjustment for exposure to tobacco and radon decay products, and a positive dose—response relationship was observed. Duration of exposure appeared to be more important than intensity in the etiology of lung cancer. The median duration of exposure was 28 years.

A preliminary case—control study of 19 lung cancer cases over the age of 55 and 141 age-matched controls was carried out among a group of underground tin miners who were exposed to ^{222}Rn and its decay products (Laurer *et al.*, 1993; see p. 91). A clear dose—response relationship was seen, with an RR of 4.7 for the highest exposure category (> 3900 pCi of skeletal ^{210}Pb at the time of last exposure to radon). Risks also increased with cumulative working-level months of exposure.

Xuan *et al.* (1993) conducted a cohort study of 17 143 employees of the Yunnan Tin Corporation; 80% of the workers were employed underground and exposed to radon. The excess RR increased linearly with exposure, rising by 0.6% per working-level month (95% CI, 0.4—0.8). Workers were also exposed to arsenic-containing dusts;

adjustment for arsenic reduced the effect of radon to 0.2% per working-level month (95% CI, 0.1−0.3).

Among male employees at the Datchang tin mine in Guangxi, mortality from lung cancer increased from 76.8/100 000 in 1973 to 178.2/100 000 in 1986. A case−control study in the area where the tin mine is located, with 69 cases and 138 controls, showed that the main risk factors for lung cancer were duration of exposure to smelting and to underground mining (Wu et al., 1989).

Haematite mining

An excess risk for lung cancer and for non-malignant respiratory disease was found among underground haematite miners in China (Chen et al., 1990); the SMR was 3.7 in comparison with nationwide male population rates. The SMR was 4.8 for people who had first been employed before mechanical ventilation and wet drilling were introduced. Workers with jobs involving heavy exposure to dust, radon and radon decay products had an SMR of 4.2. Miners with a history of silicosis had an SMR of 5.3, and those with a history of silicotuberculosis an SMR of 6.6. The risk among current smokers increased with level of exposure to dust.

Mining of several types of ore

A series of case−control studies was carried out on the basis of data from the Bulawayo (Zimbabwe) Cancer Registry, which operated during 1963−77 (Skinner et al., 1993) in an area where farming and mining were the two major economic activities. Patients were administered a questionnaire on selected cancer risk factors, including occupation, although information on occupation was missing for about 50% of cases. Male patients with cancers of the lung (877), oesophagus (826), liver (1209) and bladder (499) were compared in case−control analyses with individuals with other types of cancer. An association was found between mining and the incidence of lung cancer (odds ratio, 3.1; 95% CI, 1.07−1.60) but not of other types of cancer. The risk for lung cancer was particularly elevated among copper, gold and nickel miners, while it was not increased among coal and chromium miners and was nonsignificantly increased for asbestos miners.

Exposures to silica

Mortality from lung cancer between 1980 and 1986 was studied in a cohort of 1419 men on a Hong Kong silicosis register who had had no previous exposure to asbestos or polynuclear aromatic hydrocarbons (Ng et al., 1990). There were 28 deaths from lung cancer (SMR, 2.03; 95% CI, 1.35−2.93), all in smokers. The SMRs increased with latency and duration of exposure. Mortality from lung cancer was high among patients who had both tuberculosis and severe silicosis (SMR, 7.6, based on seven deaths).

SIRs for lung cancer were calculated for a cohort of 159 silicotics in Singapore who had worked in surface granite quarries (Chia et al., 1991). The comparison group was Chinese males in Singapore. Nine cases were found, to give an SIR of 2.01 (95% CI, 0.92−3.81); only one case was in a nonsmoker.

A cohort study was conducted on about 68 000 people employed during 1972−74 at tungsten, copper−iron and tin mines and at pottery plants in south−central China who were followed for mortality through 1989 (Chen et al., 1992; see p. 85). National rates were used to calculate expected numbers of deaths. In the overall cohort, there was no excess of mortality from cancer (SMR, 0.86; 95% CI, 0.81−0.90) or from lung cancer (SMR, 0.79; 95% CI, 0.71−0.88). The only sites at which there was a significantly increased risk for mortality from cancer were nasopharynx (SMR, 1.54) and liver (SMR, 1.15), probably due to local life-style factors and infections. Mortality from lung cancer was significantly decreased among tungsten miners and pottery workers but was close to that expected among copper−iron miners and was significantly elevated among tin miners (SMR, 1.98). No significant trend was observed in relation to estimated level of exposure to dust. The risk for lung cancer was, however, 22% higher among workers with silicosis than among those without. In a case−control study of lung cancer nested in this cohort, a significant trend for increasing risk with exposure to silica was found for tin miners but not for other miners, and a nonsignificant trend was found for pottery workers (McLaughlin *et al.*, 1992). Exposure to arsenic and polycyclic aromatic hydrocarbons was high in the tin mines.

Exposures to metals

Copper and arsenic smelting

A retrospective cohort study in China involved 18 795 workers at copper and arsenic smelters and at an ore mine (Wu, 1988). The SMR for lung cancer was 6.78 (90% CI, 5.11−8.82). An association was found between lung cancer and airborne arsenic concentration. Results of studies of lung cancer risk among Yunnan, China, tin miners exposed to radon decay products and arsenic are reported on page 117.

Iron moulding

Proportionate mortality ratios were calculated on the basis of 578 deaths among members of the South African Iron Moulders Society (Sitas *et al.*, 1989). Non-whites were excluded owing to small numbers and poor information for population comparisons. The ratio for lung cancer was increased (1.7; $p = 0.03$).

Chromate manufacture

A retrospective cohort study of 2982 workers in Chinese chromate manufacturing plants showed an increased risk for lung cancer (RR, 2.7; 90% CI, 1.3−5.5) (Wu, 1988). The latent period ranged from 2.2 to 20.3 years, with an average of 11.7 years. The excess risk was related to latency, extent of exposure and smoking habits.

Other and unspecified metal work

A case−control study in Brazil on risk factors for second cancers of the upper respiratory and digestive systems showed an elevated risk for metal workers after adjustment for tobacco and alcohol consumption (RR, 6.2; 95% CI, 1.3−30.3) (Franco *et al.*, 1991).

A case−control study involving interviews with 1249 lung cancer patients and 1345 population-based controls was conducted in Shenyang, an industrial city in northeastern China where mortality rates are high among men and women (Xu *et al.*, 1989). Employment in the nonferrous metal smelting and refining industry was associated with a smoking-adjusted increased risk for cancer among males (RR, 3.5; 95% CI, 1.6−1.8). The RR was based on 26 cases and eight controls. Most of the men had worked in the smelting industry for at least 20 years. The RR for females was 1.3 ($p > 0.05$).

A population-based study of 996 incident cases of nasopharyngeal cancer (in 718 men and 278 women) in Shanghai (Zheng *et al.*, 1992a) showed an excess incidence rate among men employed in metal smelting (11 cases; SIR, 2.25), in blacksmiths and forging press operators (56 cases; SIR, 1.36) and in metal grinders, polishers and machine tool operators (31 cases; SIR, 1.92).

Coke production, coal gasification and oil refining

A number of cohorts of workers exposed to polynuclear aromatic hydrocarbons have been studied in China (Wu, 1988). In all cases, the reference cohort was workers at a primary rolling mill. A cohort of 21 995 workers in 19 coke production plants had an SIR for lung cancer of 2.55 (90% CI, 2.13−3.03). A cohort of 3107 workers in six coal-gas plants had an SIR for lung cancer of 3.66 (90% CI, 2.36−5.43), and an excess risk was also found for digestive cancers. In a cohort of 5122 workers in two carbon plants, the SIR for lung cancer was 2.6 (90% CI, 1.79−3.6). In a cohort of 6285 workers at a shale-refining plant, increased SMRs for lung cancer (2.40; 90% CI, 1.85-3.07) and for oesophageal cancer (2.44; 1.57−3.11) were observed. In a cohort of 12 422 workers at an oil-refining plant, the only risk that was elevated was that for liver cancer (SMR, 1.99; 90% CI 1.27−2.99), which was even higher (3.88; 1.99−6.68) for workers in the fuel-oil producing department. In a cohort of 3774 workers at a synthetic oil plant, excess risks for cancers of the lung (SMR, 2.02; 90% CI, 1.34−2.93) and digestive tract (SMR, 1.56; 90% CI, 1.13−2.09) were detected.

Exposures to benzene

In a survey in China involving a sample of 20 000 workers, RRs of 5−7 for leukaemia were found among benzene-exposed workers (Goldsmith, 1985). In a survey of more than 500 000 Chinese workers exposed to benzene or mixtures containing benzene (see p. 77), 24 cases of aplastic anaemia and nine of leukaemia were found (Yin *et al.*, 1987) among people who had been exposed to benzene for between 3.5 months and 19 years. Most cases occurred among workers in shoemaking and paint production factories, where the benzene concentrations ($93−1156$ mg/m^3) were generally above the hygiene standard. The patients with aplastic anaemia had been exposed to a daily mean concentration of 1035.6 mg/m^3 benzene for an average of 118.8 days. Patients with leukaemia had been exposed for 7−25 years, except for one, who had been exposed for only two years.

A retrospective cohort study was conducted among 28 460 workers exposed to benzene in 233 factories in China (Yin *et al.*, 1989), who were compared with a cohort of 28 257 workers not exposed to benzene. SMRs for males were significantly elevated for leukaemia (5.74) and lung cancer (2.31), whereas nonsignificant elevations were observed for primary hepatocarcinoma, lymphosarcoma and cancers of the stomach, oesophagus, intestine and nasopharynx. Women showed higher SMRs than controls only for leukaemia. Benzene-exposed smokers had a mortality rate from lung cancer

2.3 times greater than that of unexposed smokers. The minimal average exposure was estimated to be 6.5 mg/m^3, and the lowest cumulative lifetime exposure to be 33.2 mg/m^3 years.

Aksoy and colleagues (1974) reported on a series of cases in an estimated population of 28 500 Turkish shoe workers who had been exposed since the 1950s to solvents and adhesives containing high levels of benzene (see p. 77). Aplastic anaemia was first observed in 1961, and 26 patients with acute leukaemia had been observed by 1967. Peak exposure levels of benzene were reported to be 30−210 ppm (96−672 mg/m^3), with rare episodes of 650 ppm (2080 mg/m^3), for periods of 1−14 years (mean, 9.7 years). The annual incidence rate of leukaemia in this group of workers was estimated to be 13/100 000, whereas that for the general population was 6/100 000.

Exposures to benzidine

The incidence of bladder cancer in benzidine-exposed workers in China is summarized in Table 3.

Table 3. Bladder cancer incidence among benzidine-exposed workers in China

Area	No. of workers	Industry	No. of cases	SIR	Comments	Reference
Various areas	2525	Benzidine-exposed workers	30	32.3	Interaction with tobacco smoking	Wu (1988)
Shanghai	736	Benzidine-based dye production	14	19.2	Excess only in presynthesis	You *et al.* (1990)
	1210	Benzidine-based dyes used in textile printing and dyeing	1	No excess		
Shanghai	901	Benzidine-based dyes used in leather tanning	6	2.73		Chen (1990)
Shanghai, Tianjin and Jilin	266	Benzidine production	9	45.7	Trend with estimated exposure; interaction with tobacco smoking	Bi *et al.* (1992)
	1271	Benzidine-based dye production	21	20.9		

SIR, standardized incidence ratio

In a retrospective cohort study of 2525 Chinese workers who had been exposed to benzidine for at least one year between 1972 and 1981, male workers had an RR of 12.9 (90% CI, 3.4−48.3) for mortality from bladder cancer and an RR of 32.2 (90% CI, 11.2−92.6) for incidence (Wu, 1988). Mortality from and the incidence of stomach and lung cancers were also slightly in excess. The study suggested a synergistic effect with cigarette smoking: the independent RR for smoking was 6.2, that for benzidine was 63.4, and that for the two exposures combined was 152.3.

Two retrospective cohort studies on bladder cancer and exposure to benzidine were conducted in Shanghai (You *et al.*, 1990). The first involved a cohort of 550 men and

186 women working in seven dyestuff factories where benzidine had served as an intermediate in the manufacture of dyes before 1976. The workers were divided in two groups: 354 assigned to presynthesis jobs and 196 to postsynthesis jobs. The SIR was 19.18 for the whole cohort and 35.00 for the presynthesis group, in which all 14 cases occurred; the SIR for the subgroup of workers assigned to transport and mixing of benzidine was 75.00. The second retrospective cohort study investigated the incidence of cancer among 1420 workers who used benzidine-derived dyes in 43 textile printing and dyeing factories. No excess of cancer was observed.

Bi *et al.* (1992) followed 1972 workers in Tianjin, Shanghai and Jilin, China, who had been exposed to benzidine (either as producers or as users in dye manufacture) between 1972 and 1981 (see p. 83). Very large excesses of mortality from (eight deaths; SMR, 17.5) and incidence of (30 cases; SIR, 25.0) bladder cancer were detected among these workers. The SIRs were 4.8 for low exposure to benzidine, 36.2 for medium exposure and 158.4 (based on eight cases) for high exposure. The risk for bladder cancer was higher among producers of benzidine (SIR, 45.7) than among users (SIR, 20.9). There was a suggestion of an interaction between exposure to benzidine and tobacco smoking, since exposed smokers had an SIR of 31.5 and nonsmokers an SIR of 11.1.

Exposure to vinyl chloride

In a cohort of 5958 Chinese workers who had been exposed to vinyl chloride for at least one year between 1958 and 1981 (see p. 83), no excess mortality was observed for any cancer (Wu, 1988).

Rubber industry

A cohort of 1624 employees at a rubber factory in Shanghai, China, were followed-up from 1972 (Zhang *et al.*, 1989). The highest SMR was observed for workers exposed to curing agents (2.86; $p < 0.05$; six cases in men and one case in women). The RR for lung cancer among smokers (after stratification by degree of exposure to curing agents and inner tubes) was 8.5 for men ($p < 0.05$) and 11.4 for women ($p < 0.05$). The RR for rubber workers exposed to curing agents or talc powder, stratified by smoking, was 3.2 for men and 4.6 for women.

A total of 8316 workers in three tyre and other rubber products manufacturing plants in Shanghai, China, were studied for cancer incidence and mortality (Chen *et al.*, 1992). Among men, the overall number of cancer cases and deaths was lower than expected (SIR, 0.78; SMR, 0.87), and there was a significant decrease in risk for cancers of the oesophagus and lung (SIR for lung cancer, 0.75); however, there was a significant increase in the risk for pancreatic cancer (SIR, 1.86). The results for bladder cancer in the whole cohort, based on 16 incident cases and eight deaths, were not statistically significant, but an increased incidence of bladder cancer was observed among workers in milling, maintenance, storage and tyre curing.

Exposure to chloromethyl methyl ether

A retrospective cohort study of 915 workers exposed to chloromethyl methyl ether and bischloromethyl ether was conducted in China (Wu, 1988). The levels of chloromethyl methyl ether in one plant ranged from 1.2 to 59 ppm in 1977–78. Between the beginning of the operations and 1981, 15 deaths from lung cancer were observed and 0.97 were expected (SMR, 15.46; 95% CI, 9.44–25.31). No association was observed between lung cancer mortality and cigarette smoking.

Textile industry

The odds ratios for nasal cancer were elevated in a case–control study among textile workers in Hong Kong (2.93 overall and 7.39 for workers with more than 15 years of employment) (Ng, 1986). In China, no elevated risk for lung cancer was found among textile workers (Levin *et al.*, 1988) or for nasopharyngeal cancer among patients who had been exposed occupationally to cotton dust (RR, 0.3; $p < 0.01$) (Yu *et al.*, 1990).

A population-based study of 996 incident cases of nasopharyngeal cancer (in 718 men and 278 women) in Shanghai (Zheng *et al.*, 1992a) showed an excess incidence among men employed as textile workers (30 cases; SIR, 1.18) and among women employed as textile weavers (23 cases; SIR, 1.64) and textile knitters (11 cases; SIR, 2.06).

Fur industry

The rate of mortality from all cancers among workers at nine fur factories in the Inner Mongolian Autonomous Region, China, was 475.6/100 000, which was higher than the rates in an iron and steel company and among non-fur workers. The rates for cancers of the oesophagus, liver and lung were particularly high (Wang, 1987).

Agriculture

Very limited information is available on cancer risks among agricultural workers in developing countries. A case–control study was carried out in Zimbabwe that involved 47 patients with bronchoscopically diagnosed cancer of the lung and 46 orthopaedic and surgical patients. Twelve of the lung cancer patients and none of the controls were tobacco farm labourers. All of the labourers smoked unprocessed tobacco (Kusemamariwo & Neill, 1990).

Five cases of mesothelioma from rural communities of India were treated in Miraj, Maharashtra, between January 1974 and March 1976 (Das *et al.*, 1976). None of the patients had been exposed to asbestos but all were involved in sugar-cane farming or an allied trade.

Time trends in mortality between 1961–71 and 1972–84 were analysed in central Luzon, the Philippines, where 80% of the heads of households are employed in rice-farming (Loevinsohn, 1987), an activity that involves intensive use of pesticides (mainly carbofuran, endrin, parathion, monocrotophos and DDT). Such use increased particularly in the second time period analysed. In men in three rural communities, mortality attributed to leukaemia increased by 480% between 1961–71 and 1972–84, from 0.6/100 000 to 3.6/100 000. The increase was greatest in the more recent years, as 7 of the 11 cases occurred between 1979 and 1984. Mortality among women remained constant. In a study of cases of cancer of the oral cavity registered in Trivandrum, Kerala, India (P. Chattopadhyay, personal communication), agricultural workers were at increased risk. The increase could not be explained by alcohol drinking or tobacco smoking or chewing. The risk was particularly high among owner cultivators, the category with the highest probable exposure to pesticides. In the same study, agricultural workers were not at increased risk for lung cancer or for cancers of the lymphohaematopoietic system.

Exposures to ionizing radiation

A follow-up study of 27 011 diagnostic X-ray workers in China showed an RR of 1.21 (95% CI, 1.08–1.35) for cancer in comparison with 25 782 physicians who did not routinely take X-rays (Wang et al., 1990). Significantly elevated risks were observed for leukaemia and for cancers of the skin, oesophagus, liver, breast, thyroid and bone.

Mixed exposures and occupations

A study of cancer incidence among male Chinese workers aged 35–64 in Singapore showed high RRs for lung cancer in bricklayers and carpenters (RR, 1.30; 95% CI, 0.92–1.83) and in transport equipment operators (1.35; 1.11–1.65), for oesophageal cancer in bricklayers and carpenters (1.63; 0.85–3.13), for skin cancer among farmers (3.22; 1.42–7.32) and for bladder cancer in machinery fitters (2.02; 0.76–5.39) (Lee, 1984).

A case–control study of 344 cases of bladder cancer and matched controls was conducted in China. The RR was 5.71 for occupational exposures to dyestuffs, rubber, cable, ink, dress pressing and cigarette manufacture and remained significant after adjustment for smoking. The RR for smoking was 1.5 (You et al., 1990). In a similar study in Shanghai, the occupations of 1219 patients with bladder cancer were compared with data from the 1982 census (Zheng et al., 1992b). Among the occupations and industries found to carry an increased risk for cancer were plastics production, textile bleaching, dyeing and finishing, metalwork, petroleum refining, railway engine drivers and firemen and paper processing. A case–control study on bladder cancer in Argentina showed high risks for truck and railway drivers (4.31) and oil refinery workers (6.22); the associations persisted after adjustment for tobacco smoking (Iscovich et al., 1987). No association with occupation was observed in a case–control study of Hodgkin's disease in Brazil (Kirchhoff et al., 1980). A case–control study in Uruguay showed an RR of 2.8 (95% CI, 1.1–7.6) for oropharyngeal cancers in bricklayers (adjusted for tobacco and alcohol consumption) and an RR of 4.9 (95% CI, 1.2–19.4) for laryngeal cancer in drivers (Oreggia et al., 1989).

Occupational risk factors for 13 489 cases of gastric cancer were studied in China on the basis of data from the Shanghai Cancer Registry. Several occupations were found to be associated with statistically significant increases in risk; the most notable were grain farming (SIR, 4.02) and several jobs involving potential exposure to metal, wood and textile dusts and to fossil combustion products. These included elevated SIRs for wood sawyers, plywood makers (1.76), cabinetmakers (1.47), other wood and bamboo workers (1.95), blacksmiths (1.56), metal grinders (1.41) and sheet metal workers (1.40). The SIRs for nurses, pesticide production workers and petroleum refinery workers were more than four times greater than expected, although the numbers of cases were small. The only occupations associated with significantly elevated risks and in which at least five cases occurred among women were plastics and plastic products manufacture (41 cases; SIR, 1.60), knitting (1.48) and weaving (1.17) (Kneller *et al.*, 1990).

A study of lung cancer in China recorded histories of occupational exposure to pitch-tar compounds, asbestos, nickel, chromium, arsenic, beryllium, cadmium, lead, zinc, wood dust, nitrosamines, radiation and mustard gas. The authors calculated mortality rates by city and found the highest rates for cities where the main industries are machinery and metallurgical processing, and petroleum and chemical factories. These were also the largest cities (Xiao & Xu, 1985).

Occupation was evaluated as a potential risk factor for lung cancer in a large population-based case−control study in Shanghai, which involved 773 male cases and 760 controls and 672 female cases and 735 controls. Occupational and smoking histories were obtained by interview. Significantly raised risks were detected among men in farming (odds ratio, 1.6) and agricultural production (1.6). Elevated but not statistically significant excess risks were found for chemical industry workers (1.7) and for exposures to wool and coal dusts, smoke from burning fuels and chemicals fumes. A decreased risk was observed for textile industry workers (0.7; 95% CI, 0.5−1.0). The highest risk among chemical industry workers was found for individuals ever employed in the making of soaps, detergents, perfumes and cosmetics (3.2; 95% CI, 1.0−10.2). No unusual risk was observed for rubber and plastic products manufacture (Levin *et al.*, 1988).

No excess risk for any cancer was observed in a study of taxi drivers in Singapore (Koh *et al.*, 1988). In a case−control study of 306 cases in China, any occupational exposure to products of combustion was found to be related to risk for nasopharyngeal carcinoma (RR, 2.4; $p < 0.001$). The types of combustion products named by the 63 patients and 33 controls were those associated with welding (15 cases, 8 controls), coal and coke burning (20 cases, 10 controls), burning of liquid fuels (16 cases, 9 controls) and others (17 cases, 11 controls). Adjustment for use of tobacco and other confounders in a logistic regression model did not change the risk. The risk for exposure for more than 10 years was 9 (95% CI, 2.8−28.8) (Yu *et al.*, 1990).

A case−control study of 60 incident cases of cancer of the nasal cavity and sinuses and 414 controls was conducted in Shanghai (Zheng *et al.*, 1992c). Occupational exposures to wood and silica dusts and to petroleum products were associated with moderate increases in risk.

A case−control study of 120 cases of nasopharyngeal cancer in northeastern Thailand (Sriamporn *et al.*, 1992) showed an elevated risk for agricultural workers (RR, 2.8; 95% CI, 1.3−6.2) and a stronger risk for agricultural workers involved in woodcutting (8.0; 2.3−28.2).

Several case−control studies of nasopharyngeal cancer, in Malaysia (Armstrong *et al.*, 1983) and China (Lin *et al.*, 1973; Henderson *et al.*, 1976; Yu *et al.*, 1986), reported elevated risks associated with nonspecific exposures to dust, but the information on exposure was not sufficiently detailed to allow further conclusions to be drawn.

References

Aksoy, M., Erdem, S. & Dinçol, G. (1974) Leukemia in shoeworkers exposed chronically to benzene. *Blood*, **44**, 837−841

Armstrong, R.W., Armstrong, M.J., Yu, M.C. & Henderson, B.E. (1983) Salted fish and inhalants as risk factors for nasopharyngeal carcinoma in Malaysian Chinese. *Cancer Res.*, 43, 2967–2970

Bi, W., Hayes, R.B., Feng, P., Qi, Y., You, X., Zhen, J., Zhang, M., Qu, B., Fu, Z., Chen, M., Co Chien, H.T. & Blot, W.J. (1992) Mortality and incidence of bladder cancer in benzidine-exposed workers in China. *Am. J. Ind. Med.*, 21, 481–489

Botha, J.L., Irwig, L.M. & Strebel, P.M. (1986) Excess mortality from stomach cancer, lung cancer, and asbestosis and/or mesothelioma in crocidolite mining districts in South Africa. *Am. J. Epidemiol.*, 123, 30–40

Bradshaw, E., McGlashan, N.D., Fitzgerald, D. & Harington, J.S. (1982) Analyses of cancer incidence in black gold miners from southern Africa (1964–79). *Br. J. Cancer*, 46, 737–748

Chen, J.-G. (1990) A cohort study on the cancer experience among workers exposed to benzidine-derived dyes in Shanghai leather-tanning industry. *Chin. J. Prev. Med.*, 24, 328–331 (in Chinese)

Chen, S.Y., Hayes, R.B., Liang, S.R., Li, Q.G., Stewart, P.A. & Blair, A. (1990) Mortality experience of haematite mine workers in China. *Br. J. Ind. Med.*, 47, 175–181

Chen, J., McLaughlin, J.K., Zhang, J.-Y., Stone, B.J., Luo, J., Chen, R.-A., Dosemeci, M., Rexing, S.H., Wu, Z., Hearl, F.J., McCawley, M.A. & Blot, W.J. (1992) Mortality among dust-exposed Chinese mine and pottery workers. *J. Occup. Med.*, 34, 311–316

Cheng, W.-N. & Kong, J. (1992) A retrospective mortality cohort study of chrysotile asbestos products workers in Tianjin 1972–1987. *Environ. Res.*, 59, 271–278

Chia, S.-E., Chia, K.-S., Phoon, W.-H. & Lee, H.-P. (1991) Silicosis and lung cancer among Chinese granite workers. *Scand. J. Work Environ. Health*, 17, 170–174

Cullen, M.R. & Baloyi, R.S. (1991) Chrysotile asbestos and health in Zimbabwe: I. Analysis of miners and millers compensated for asbestos-related diseases since independence (1980). *Am. J. Ind. Med.*, 19, 161–169

Das, P.B., Fletcher, A.G., Jr & Deodhare, S.G. (1976) Mesothelioma in an agricultural community in India: a clinicopathological study. *Aust. N.Z. J. Surg.*, 46, 218–226

Franco, E.L., Kowalski, L.P. & Kanda, J.L. (1991) Risk factors for second cancers of the upper respiratory and digestive systems: a case–control study. *J. Clin. Epidemiol.*, 44, 615–625

Goldsmith, J.R. (1985) Occupational health in Chinese metallurgical industries: report based on a visit. *Am. J. Ind. Med.*, 7, 353–357

Henderson, B.E., Louie, E., Jing, J.S.H., Buell, P. & Gardner, M.B. (1976) Risk factors associated with nasopharyngeal carcinoma. *New Engl. J. Med.*, 295, 1101–1106

Hessel, P.A., Sluis-Cremer, G.K. & Hnizdo, E. (1986) Case–control study of silicosis, silica exposure, and lung cancer in white South African gold miners. *Am. J. Ind. Med.*, 10, 57–62

Hnizdo, E., Sluis-Cremer, G.K. & Abramowitz, J.A. (1991) Emphysema type in relation to silica dust exposure in South African gold miners. *Am. Rev. Respir. Dis.*, 143, 1241–1247

Ho, S.F., Lee, H.P. & Phoon, W.H. (1987) Malignant mesothelioma in Singapore. *Br. J. Ind. Med.*, 44, 788–789

Iscovich, J., Castelletto, R., Estève, J., Muñoz, N., Colanzi, R., Coronel, A., Deamezola, I., Tassi, V. & Arslan, A. (1987) Tobacco smoking, occupational exposure and bladder cancer in Argentina. *Int. J. Cancer*, 40, 734–740

Kirchhoff, L.V., Evans, A.S., McClelland, K.E., Carvalho, R.P.S. & Pannuti, C.S. (1980) A case–control study of Hodgkin's disease in Brazil. I. Epidemiological aspects. *Am. J. Epidemiol.*, 112, 595–608

Kneller, R.W., Gao, Y.-T., McLaughlin, J.K., Gao, R.-N., Blot, W.J., Liu, M.-H., Sheng, J.-P. & Fraumeni, J.F., Jr (1990) Occupational risk factors for gastric cancer in Shanghai, China. *Am. J. Ind. Med.*, 18, 69–78

Koh, D., Guanco-Chua, S. & Ong, C.N. (1988) A study of the mortality patterns of taxi drivers in Singapore. *Ann. Acad. Med.*, 17, 579–582

Kusemamariwo, T. & Neill, P. (1990) Carcinoma of the bronchus in tobacco farm workers. An unrecognised high risk group. *Trop. Geogr. Med.*, 42, 261–264

Lam, W.K., Kung, T.M., Ma, P.L., So, S.Y. & Mok, C.K. (1983) First report of asbestos-related diseases in Hong Kong. *Trop. Geogr. Med.*, 35, 225–229

Laurer, G.R., Gang, Q.T., Lubin, J.H., Huna-Yao, L., Kan, C.S., Xiang, Y.S., Jian, C.Z., Yi, H., De, G.W. & Blot, W.J. (1993) Skeletal ^{210}Pb levels and lung cancer among radon-exposed tin miners in southern China. *Health Phys.*, **64**, 253–259

Lee, H.P. (1984) Cancer incidence in Singapore by occupational groups. *Ann. Acad. Med.*, **13** (Suppl.), 366–370

Levin, L.I., Zheng, W., Blot, W.J., Gao, Y.-T. & Fraumeni, J.F., Jr (1988) Occupation and lung cancer in Shanghai: a case–control study. *Br. J. Ind. Med.*, **45**, 450–458

Lin, T.M., Chen, K.P., Lin, C.C., Hsu, M.N., Tu, S.M., Chiang, T.C., Jung, P.F. & Hirayama, T. (1973) Retrospective study on nasopharyngeal cancer. *J. Natl Cancer Inst.*, **51**, 1403–1408

Loevinsohn, M.E. (1987) Insecticide use and increased mortality in rural Central Luzon, Philippines. *Lancet*, **i**, 1359–1362

McGlashan, N.D., Harington, J.S. & Bradshaw, E. (1982) Eleven sites of cancer in black gold miners from southern Africa: a geographic enquiry. *Br. J. Cancer*, **46**, 947–954

McLaughlin, J.K., Chen, J.-Q., Dosemeci, M., Chen, R.-A., Rexing, S.H., Wu, Z., Hearl, F.J., McCawley, M.A. & Blot, W.J. (1992) A nested case–control study of lung cancer among silica exposed workers in China. *Br. J. Ind. Med.*, **49**, 167–171

Méndez Vargas, M.M., Torres, L.M., Stanislawski, E.C. & Mendoza Ugalde, H.A. (1982) Malignant mesothelioma in an asbestos worker. *Rev. Méd. Inst. Mex. Seg. Soc.*, **20**, 249–257 (in Spanish)

Mostert, C. & Meintjes, R. (1979) Asbestosis and mesothelioma on the Rhodesia railways. *Centr. Afr. J. Med.*, **25**, 72–74

Ng, T.P. (1986) A case–referent study of cancer of the nasal cavity and sinuses in Hong Kong. *Int. J. Epidemiol.*, **15**, 171–175

Ng, T.P., Chan, S.L. & Lee, J. (1990) Mortality of a cohort of men in a silicosis register: further evidence of an association with lung cancer. *Am. J. Ind. Med.*, **17**, 163–171

Oreggia, F., de Stefani, E., Correa, P., Rivero, S., Fernandez, G., Leiva, J. & Zavala, D. (1989) Occupational exposure in cancer of the oral cavity, pharynx and larynx. *Anal. O.R.L. Iber.-Am.*, **16**, 365–376 (in Spanish)

Osburn, H.S. (1957) Cancer of the lung in Gwandi. *Centr. Afr. J. Med.*, **3**, 215–223

Qiao, Y.-L., Taylor, P.R., Yao, S.-X., Schatzkin, A., Mao, B.-L., Lubin, J., Rao, J.-Y., McAdams, M., Xuan, X.-Z. & Li, J.-Y. (1989) Relation of radon exposure and tobacco use to lung cancer among tin miners in Yunnan Province, China. *Am. J. Ind. Med.*, **16**, 511–521

Sitas, F., Douglas, A.J. & Webster, E.C. (1989) Respiratory disease mortality patterns among South African iron moulders. *Br. J. Ind. Med.*, **46**, 310–315

Skinner, M.E.G., Parkin, D.M., Vizcaino, A.P. & Ndhlovu, A. (1993) *Cancer in the African Population of Bulawayo, Zimbabwe, 1963–1977* (IARC Technical Report No. 15), Lyon, IARC

Solomons, K. (1984) Malignant mesothelioma — clinical and epidemiological features. A report of 80 cases. *S. Afr. Med. J.*, **66**, 407–412

Sriamporn, S., Vatanasapt, V., Pisani, P., Yongchaiyudha, S. & Rungpitarangsri, V. (1992) Environmental risk factors for nasopharyngeal cancer: a case–control study in northeastern Thailand. *Cancer Epidemiol. Biomarkers Prev.*, **1**, 345–348

Sun, S.-Q. (1988) Etiology of lung cancer at the Gejiu tin mine, China. In: Miller, R.W., Watanabe, S., Fraumeni, J.F., Jr, Sugimura, T., Takayama, S. & Sugano, H., eds, *Unusual Occurrences as Clues to Cancer Etiology*, Tokyo, Japan Scientific Societies Press/London, Taylor & Francis Ltd, pp. 103–115

Talent, J.M., Harrison, W.O., Solomon, A. & Webster, I. (1980) A survey of black mineworkers of the Cape crocidolite mines. In: Wagner, J.C., ed., *Biological Effects of Mineral Fibres*, Vol. 2 (IARC Scientific Publications No. 30), Lyon, IARC, pp. 723–729

Taylor, P.R., Qiao, Y.-L., Schatzkin, A., Yao, S.-X., Lubin, J., Mao, B.-L., Rao, J.-Y., McAdams, M., Xuan, X.-Z. & Li, J.-Y. (1989) Relation of arsenic exposure to lung cancer among tin miners in Yunnan Province, China. *Br. J. Ind. Med.*, **46**, 881–886

Wagner, J.C. (1991) The discovery of the association between blue asbestos and mesotheliomas and the aftermath. *Br. J. Ind. Med.*, **48**, 399–403

Wagner, J.C., Sleggs, C.A. & Marchand, P. (1960) Diffuse pleural mesothelioma and asbestos exposure in the north western Cape Province. *Br. J. Ind. Med.*, **17**, 260–271

Wang, H.-L. (1987) Cancer among fur workers. *Chung Hua Fang I Hsueh Tsa Chih*, 21, 129–132

Wang, J.-X., Inskip, P.D., Boice, J.D., Jr, Li, B.-X., Zhang, J.-Y. & Fraumeni, J.F., Jr (1990) Cancer incidence among medical diagnostic X-ray workers in China, 1950 to 1985. *Int. J. Cancer*, 45, 889–895

Wu, W. (1988) Occupational cancer epidemiology in the People's Republic of China. *J. Occup. Med.*, 30, 968–974

Wu, K.-G., Fu, H., Mo, C.-Z. & Yu, L.-Z. (1989) Smelting, underground mining, smoking, and lung cancer: a case–control study in a tin mine area. *Biomed. Environ. Sci.*, 2, 98–105

Wyndham, C.H., Bezuidenhout, B.N., Greenacre, M.J. & Sluis-Cremer, G.K. (1986) Mortality of middle-aged white South African goldminers. *Br. J. Ind. Med.*, 43, 677–684

Xiao, H.-P. & Xu, Z.-Y. (1985) Air pollution and lung cancer in Liaoning Province, People's Republic of China. *Natl Cancer Inst. Monogr.*, 69, 53–58

Xu, Z.-Y., Blot, W.J., Xiao, H.-P., Wu, A., Feng, Y.-P., Stone, B.J., Sun, J., Ershow, A.G., Henderson, B.E. & Fraumeni, J.F., Jr (1989) Smoking, air pollution, and the high rates of lung cancer in Shenyang, China. *J. Natl Cancer Inst.*, 81, 1800–1806

Xuan, X.-Z., Schatzkin, A., Mao, B.-L., Taylor, P.R., Li, J.-Y., Tangrea, J., Yao, S.-X., Qiao, Y.-L., Giffen, C. & McAdams, M. (1991) Feasibility of conducting a lung-cancer chemoprevention trial among tin miners in Yunnan, P.R. China. *Cancer Causes Control*, 2, 175–182

Xuan, X.Z., Lubin, J.H., Li, J.Y., Yang, L.F., Luo, A.S., Lan, Y., Wang, J.Z. & Blot, W.J. (1993) A cohort study in southern China of tin miners exposed to radon and radon decay products. *Health Phys.*, 64, 120–131

Yang, M.-D., Wang, J.-D., Wang, Y.-L., Guo, P.-S., Yao, Z.-Q., Lu, P.-L., Gu, X.-Y., Dong, Y.-L., Lu, M.-X., Zhu, P., Yan, S.-G., Liu, Q.-P., Jiang, M.-C., Chen, Z.-Q., Fang, S.-Q., Ren, S.-Y., Shen, D., Qiao, T.-Y., Huang, F.-S. & Jiang, Z.-D. (1985) Changes in health conditions in the Huainan coal mine in the past three decades. *Scand. J. Work Environ. Health*, 11 (Suppl. 4), 64–67

Yin, S.-N., Li, Q., Liu, Y., Tian, F., Du, C. & Jin, C. (1987) Occupational exposure to benzene in China. *Br. J. Ind. Med.*, 44, 192–195

Yin, S.-N., Li, G.-L., Tain, F.-D., Fu, Z.-I., Jin, C., Chen, Y.-J., Luo, S.-J., Ye, P.-Z., Zhang, J.-Z., Wang, G.-C., Zhang, X.-C., Wu, H.-N. & Zhong, Q.-C. (1989) A retrospective cohort study of leukemia and other cancers in benzene workers. *Environ. Health Perspectives*, 82, 207–213

You, X.-Y., Chen, J.-G. & Hu, Y.-N. (1990) Studies on the relation between bladder cancer and benzidine or its derived dyes in Shanghai. *Br. J. Ind. Med.*, 47, 544–552

Yu, M.C., Ho, J.H.C., Lai, S.-H. & Henderson, B.E. (1986) Cantonese-style salted fish as a cause of nasopharyngeal carcinoma: report of a case–control study in Hong Kong. *Cancer Res.*, 46, 956–961

Yu, M.C., Garabrant, D.H., Huang, T.-B. & Henderson, B.E. (1990) Occupational and other non-dietary risk factors for nasopharyngeal carcinoma in Guangzhou, China. *Int. J. Cancer*, 45, 1033–1039

Zhang, Z.-F., Yu, S.-Z., Li, W.-X. & Choi, B.C.K. (1989) Smoking, occupational exposure to rubber, and lung cancer. *Br. J. Ind. Med.*, 46, 12–15

Zheng, W., McLaughlin, J.K., Gao, Y.T., Gao, R.N. & Blot, W.J. (1992a) Occupational risks for nasopharyngeal cancer in Shanghai. *J. Occup. Med.*, 34, 1004–1007

Zheng, W., McLaughlin, J.K., Gao, Y.T., Silverman, D.T., Gao, R.N. & Blot, W.J. (1992b) Bladder cancer and occupation in Shanghai, 1980–1984. *Am. J. Ind. Med.*, 21, 877–885

Zheng, W., Blot, W.J., Shu, X.-O., Diamond, E.L., Gao, Y.-T., Ji, B.-T. & Fraumeni, J.F., Jr (1992c) A population-based case–control study of cancers of the nasal cavity and paranasal sinuses in Shanghai. *Int. J. Cancer*, 52, 557–561

Zwi, A.B., Reid, G., Landau, S.P., Kielkowski, D., Sitas, F. & Becklake, M.R. (1989) Mesothelioma in South Africa, 1976–84: incidence and case characteristics. *Int. J. Epidemiol.*, 18, 320–329

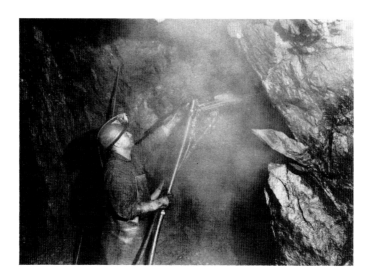

Above: Silicosis is a major hazard in mining because of heavy exposure to silica dust. In this Chilean copper mine, a 'wet' drill is now used to reduce dust levels.

Photo by P. Larsen, courtesy of World Health Organization

Below: Exposure to fibres and to solvents occurs in work on fibreglass products, as in this small factory in Papua New Guinea.

Photo: Courtesy of the International Labour Office

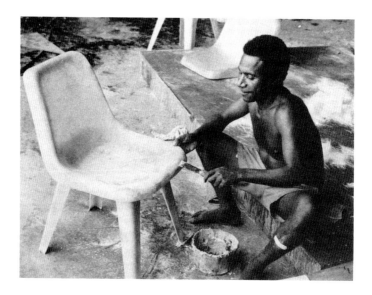

Chapter 8. Other Diseases

E. Matos and P. Boffetta

Occupational carcinogens often also cause diseases other than cancer. These diseases are important in the context of this review, not only because they may represent significant morbidity in themselves, but also because the occurrence of such diseases may indicate the presence of significant exposure to occupational carcinogens. In this chapter, we review evidence relating to asbestosis, silicosis and blood disorders and briefly discuss other diseases caused by occupational carcinogens in developing countries.

Asbestosis

Exposure to asbestos causes a number of lung disorders other than lung carcinoma and mesothelioma, including fibrosis (asbestosis), pleural fibrosis and plaques. Studies in which the prevalence of asbestosis in developing countries was reported or mentioned are summarized in Table 1. Many of the studies do not refer to the number of workers surveyed, and some prevalence figures are based on populations that are not representative of all workers in the country. Nevertheless, a higher prevalence is consistently observed among workers with longer duration of exposure. Table 1 is complemented by data in Table 2 in which permissible exposure levels for asbestos, numbers of exposed workers and information on asbestosis, mesothelioma and lung cancer are shown by country. Asbestosis is recognized as an occupational disease in 17 of the 32 countries surveyed, but information on the number of cases is seldom available. In addition to asbestosis, seven countries recognize both lung cancer and mesothelioma as occupational diseases, and four recognize neither of them. Cameroon and Peru recognize asbestosis and lung cancer but not mesothelioma; Cyprus recognizes asbestosis and mesothelioma but not lung cancer; and Botswana recognizes only mesothelioma. Five countries do not recognize any of these diseases. These issues are discussed further in Chapter 9.

Official figures may underestimate the true incidence of asbestos-related diseases in South Africa. A total of 21 665 miners were working in the asbestos mines in 1977; of these, 91.6% were black. Of the notified cases of asbestos-related disease, 43% were in white workers and 57% in blacks. The authors stated that there could be underreporting of cases in black workers owing to lack of follow-up of workers, the infrequent availability of diagnostic and technical means for identifying the long-term effects of exposure, and diagnosis in the country of origin of migrants who return home after they develop an asbestos-related disease (Myers, 1981; Myers *et al.*, 1985; Packard, 1989).

E. Matos & P. Boffetta

Table 1. Prevalence of asbestosis in selected industries in developing countries

Country	Industry/occupation	Year of survey	Prevalence (%)	No. of workers studied	Remarks	References
China	Textile and friction products	1980	20.0	NR	Highest prevalence in small plants	Christiani & Gu (1988)
Egypt	Asbestos–cement, > 20 years' exposure	1969	81.0	NR		Scansetti et al. (1975)
India	NR	NR	7.0–9.0	NR		El Batawi (1986)
Kenya	Five uses of asbestos	NR	2.6	700	13/18 workers had intermittent exposure	Sakari (1990)
Kuwait	Asbestos–cement	1990	0.32	NR		Mohamed (1990)
South Africa	Crocidolite/amosite mines/mills	1979		1962		Irwig et al. (1979)
	All workers		7.6[a] / 7.3[b]			
	> 20 years' exposure		33.6[a] / 26.7[b]			
	Asbestos mines and non-mining industries	1970 and 1977	71.5–79	NR		Baloyi (1989)
Swaziland	Ship stevedores > 15 years' exposure	1985	30.0 / 40.0	203		Myers et al. (1985)
	Chrysotile mines/mills	1982	30.0	224		McDermott et al. (1982)
Zimbabwe	Mines	1963–67	0.5	7000		Baloyi (1989)

NR, not reported
[a] Prevalence of pleural abnormalities
[b] Prevalence of parenchymal abnormalities

Table 2. Permissible exposure levels, numbers of exposed workers, and recognition of chronic diseases causally associated with exposure to asbestos in developing countries

Country or region	PEL (f/ml)	No. of exposed workers[a]	Asbestosis	Mesothelioma	Lung cancer	Reference
Angola	No	1000	No	No	No	IARC survey
Argentina	2					Cook (1987)
Botswana	No	100	No	Yes	No	IARC survey
Brazil	2	20–30 000	Yes	No	No	IARC survey
Cameroon	No	NR	Yes	No	Yes	IARC survey
Chile	2					Cook (1987)
China	2					Ng (1986)
Colombia	2		Yes	Yes	Yes	Colombian Government (1987)
Cuba	1	2200	Yes	No	No	IARC survey
Cyprus	0.1–2[b]	330	Yes	Yes	No	IARC survey
Costa Rica	No	NR	No	No	No	IARC survey
Egypt	2	NR	Yes	Yes	Yes	IARC survey
Ethiopia	No	NR	No	No	No	IARC survey
Jordan	No	200	No	No	No	IARC survey
Hong Kong	No		Yes			Government of Hong Kong (1987)
Kuwait	2	425	Yes	Yes	Yes	IARC survey
India	0.2–2[b]	9900	Yes	Yes	Yes	IARC survey
Indonesia	1					ILO (1984)
Mexico	2					Cook (1987)
Mongolia	No		No	No		IARC survey
Morocco	No	1300	Yes	No	No	IARC survey
Nigeria	2b	NR	Yes	No	No	IARC survey
Peru	No	600	Yes	No	Yes	IARC survey
Philippines	2	NR	Yes	c	c	IARC survey
Republic of Korea	Yes					Cook (1987)
Singapore	0.2–2[b]	2596				Chia et al. (1991)
South Africa	5	10 724[d]	Yes	Yes	Yes	Myers (1981); Solomons (1984)
Thailand	5b	2000	Yes	Yes	Yes	IARC survey
Turkey	No	2500	Yes	Yes	Yes	IARC survey
Venezuela	0.5					Cook (1987)
Zambia	0.2–1[b]					IARC survey
Zimbabwe	2		Yes			Baloyi (1989); Cullen & Baloyi (1991)

PEL, permissible exposure level; f, fibres; No, no PEL or legislation exists; Yes, asbestos is included in the list of carcinogens but no PEL is given; blank, no information was available; NR, not reported

[a] Based on the IARC survey; probably underestimates

[b] The first or the only figure corresponds to the PEL for crocidolite fibres; from ILO (1984)

[c] 74 cases of cancer (site unspecified) were recognized by the Employees' Compensation Commission (January–November 1991)

[d] From Solomons (1984)

In white and mixed-race workers in crocidolite and amosite mines and mills in South Africa, the prevalence of parenchymal but not pleural abnormalities was significantly predicted by fibre concentration after taking into account the effects of age and duration of exposure, but not by race or asbestos type (Irwig et al., 1979).

Lung function and radiographical indices of exposure to chrysotile asbestos were investigated in 438 of 2100 workers at the Havelock mines in Swaziland, which had been in activity since the late 1930s. Estimated annual decline in lung function and the rate of progression of pneumoconiosis were doubled in workers in grading and bagging sections of the mill, where exposure was heaviest (McDermott et al., 1982).

In Zimbabwe, 27 of about 300 men certified by the Pneumoconiosis Bureau as having occupational lung disease after 1984 had findings consistent with one or more asbestos-associated diseases: 21 men had radiographical and/or pathological evidence of asbestosis, and 18 of these had been exposed exclusively in mines and/or mills. Three of the patients died from probable malignancies (one confirmed mesothelioma) and five from respiratory failure and/or cor pulmonale. The 10 who survived generally had severe disease, as judged radiographically. The exposures of the patients had usually been long, ranging from 17 to 37 years with a mean of 22.3. The latency prior to recognition of disease was comparable (range, 17–42 years; mean, 27.2) (Cullen & Baloyi, 1991). A dose–response relationship between exposure to asbestos and functional lung loss was reported (Cullen et al., 1991).

Cases of asbestosis were described in Kenya and in Sri Lanka among workers involved in lagging and delagging boilers (Uragoda et al., 1983; Kurppa et al., 1984); another case was reported in Kuwait among workers in an asbestos-pipe factory (Mohamed, 1990). A survey was conducted in Kenya of 700 workers involved in all five major plants where asbestos was used. Only 18 of the workers had characteristics of asbestosis, and 13 of these were from a metal factory where they had intermittent exposure. No other respiratory disorder, such as pleural plaques, was seen (Sakari, 1990).

In spite of the fact that asbestos is mined and used extensively in India (see Chapter 5), only one study has been reported of exposed workers, which involved 22 workers at an asbestos–cement factory. The sister chromatid exchange rate and the number of chromosomal aberrations (chromatid gaps and breaks) were statistically significantly increased over that in an unexposed population (Fatma et al., 1991).

Thus, permissible exposure levels sometimes exist in developing countries, but the authorities are either not aware of such levels or have no information on the relationship between asbestos and disease. Furthermore, no reliable data are available in most countries on the number of workers exposed: In relation to the estimated amount of asbestos used or mined, the reported numbers are generally underestimates of the real situation. Very little epidemiological research has been carried out, and the real incidence and prevalence of asbestos-related diseases in the majority of developing countries are difficult to determine.

Silicosis

Silicosis is an occupational disease that results from accumulation of silica dust in the lungs and reaction of the tissues to its presence. Associations between silicosis and lung cancer after occupational exposure to dust containing crystalline silica have been observed among miners, quarry workers, foundry workers, ceramic workers, granite workers and stone cutters (IARC, 1987).

Silicosis is recognized as a major health problem in copper and tin mines in South America, in gold and copper mines in Africa, among lead, zinc, gold and mica miners and slate-pencil workers in India and in gold, copper, uranium, sulfur and coal mines in China. Granite quarrying is undertaken in many countries, and high prevalences of silicosis have been reported in quarriers in Singapore, Malaysia and Hong Kong (Ng, 1992).

The prevalence rates of silicosis among workers in developing countries are summarized in Table 3. Some of the studies in which the prevalence of silicosis was estimated include a considerable number of workers, such as a nationwide survey of nearly 3 million people in China, a survey of 40 000 workers in the Republic of Korea and the studies in Bolivia; other studies include smaller numbers of workers. Information stratified by duration of exposure is seldom available, but when it is (stone cutters in India, several exposures in South Africa and Zimbabwe) a consistent increase is seen with years of exposure. Comparisons between countries are difficult, however, because the industries in which the exposures occur are different. The two studies of haematite miners (in China and Egypt) show a prevalence of silicosis of about 25%. Estimates for ceramics and pottery workers vary, ranging from 1.8% in Egypt to 76.7% in Brazil (the latter based on 76 workers). In the IARC survey (see Appendix), only four countries provided numbers of reported cases of silicosis: India, 1239 cases in 1949–89; Mongolia, 841 cases in 1981–91; Thailand, two cases in 1977–89; and Turkey, nine cases in 1990.

Additional information is worth mentioning. In Chile, 844 new cases of pneumoconiosis (mainly silicosis) were notified for the whole country in 1982; pneumoconiosis rates of 489 and 580 per 100 000 total working population were estimated for the regions where the mines are located (Prenafeta, 1984). In a survey of 54 workers involved in quarrying, drying and/or calcining, packaging and storing diatomaceous earth in Kenya (Sakari, 1990), 27 were found to have silicosis at various stages. In a survey of 806 copper miners in Uganda in 1960, 54 were found to be silicotic (Ogaram, 1990).

The Anshan Iron and Steel Company in China began operation in 1951. In the sintering plant, which employed 5000 workers, 219 cases of silicosis were identified. The concentration of silica in air in 1983 was lower than the standard of 10 mg/m^3 in 79% of samples (Goldsmith, 1985). The National Center for Occupational Health in South Africa registered 217 cases of silicosis between 1972 and 1986, 50% of which were observed in foundries and 30% in ceramics factories, refractories and ore and stone crushing works (Ehrlich *et al.*, 1988). Six cases of silicosis were described among gemstone workers in South Africa, and the silica content of samples of dust taken in one of two lapidaries operating in the Western Cape was 79–81%; no fibre was present (White *et al.*, 1991).

In a survey of 219 quarry workers in Singapore (Ng *et al.*, 1992), 12.5% of highly exposed drilling and crushing workers were found to have silicosis in comparison with

Table 3. Prevalence of silicosis in selected industries in developing countries and regions

Country or region	Industry/occupation	Year of survey	Prevalence (%)	No. of workers studied	Remarks	References
Bolivia	Mines (tin)	1964–68	22.2	24 955		Pinell (1976)
	Mines (unspecified)	1981	7.6	7 600		El Batawi (1986)
	Mines (tin)	1985	40.0	8 500	Includes silicotuberculosis	Michaels et al. (1985)
Brazil	Ceramics	1981	76.7	76	Highest exposure in melting section	Nogueira et al. (1981)
Chile	Mines	1981	21.4[a]	NR		Prenafeta (1984)
China	Mines (haematite)	1989	25.0	5 406		Chen et al. (1990)
	Several industries	1974–76	3.1	2 900 000	Survey by chest radiography	Gu (1985)
	Metallurgy		5.5	NR		
	Construction		1.7	NR		
Colombia	Mines (coal)	1985	15.0[a]	NR		Michaels et al. (1985)
Egypt	Mines (phosphate)	1979	43.3	605		Noweir (1986)
	Refractory materials	1979	33.0	1 197		
	Mines (haematite)	1979	24.6	1 292		
	Foundries	1979	12.9	379		
	Steel mills	1979	7.1	381		
	Ceramics and china	1979	1.8	766		
Hong Kong	Granite quarries	1983–85	8.0	776	Preparation of ore	Ng & O'Kelly (1987)
	Site-formation and crushing		12.0	208		
	Caisson workers		15.0	135		
India	Mines (mica)	1959	32.1	329		Ng (1992)
	Metal grinding	1959	27.2	44		
	Refractory bricks	1959	21.1	327		
	Pottery	1959	15.7	808		
	Slate pencil manufacture	1985	54.6	593		Saiyed et al. (1985)
	Stone cutting	1972	35.2	227		Gupta et al. (1972)
	< 16 years' exposure		23.0	174		
	> 16 years' exposure		75.5	40		

Table 3 (contd)

Country or region	Industry/occupation	Year of survey	Prevalence (%)	No. of workers studied	Remarks	References
Malaysia	Granite quarries	1976	25.0	226	Exposure > 5 years	Singh (1977)
	5–9 years' exposure		9.0	NR		
	≥ 20 years' exposure		32.0	NR		
Nicaragua	Mines (gold)	1990	1.2	824	Most heavily exposed	Aragón et al. (1990)
Philippines	Mines, ceramics, glass manufacture, cement	1989	7.5–17.5	NR	Survey of industries with potential exposure to silica dust	N.S. Chipongian (personal communication)
Republic of Korea	Mines (unspecified)	1981	3.5	4 107		El Batawi (1986)
	Mines (coal)	1976	3.4	40 000	Medical surveillance	Ng (1992)
	Mines (metal ore)	1976	0.9	1 840		
Singapore	Granite quarries	1971	15.0	1 230		Ng et al. (1992)
South Africa	Ferrous foundries	1988	7.3	551		Ehrlich et al. (1988)
	> 20 years' exposure		28.7	NR		
	Pottery	1991	3.9	358		Rees & Kielkowski (1991)
	> 20 years' exposure		31.8	NR		
	Bricks	1991	4.4	268		
	> 20 years' exposure		17.4	NR		
	Refractory ceramics	1991	5.5	491		
	> 20 years' exposure		6.8	NR		
Sri Lanka	Mines (underground)	1987	3.4[a]	340		Uragoda (1989)
Sudan	Chromite ores	1988	18.2	77		Ballal (1986)
Zimbabwe	Mines (coal, nickel, copper and gold)	1990	6.0[a]	725		Cullen & Baloyi (1990)
	≥ 20 years' exposure		20.0[a]	NR		

NR, not reported

[a] Prevalence of pneumoconiosis

0.8% of maintenance and transportation workers with low exposure. No case of silicosis was found in quarry workers first exposed after 1979, and it was concluded that the control measures introduced in 1972−79 had been successful.

Blood disorders

The prevalence of leukopenia (< 4000/mm^3 white blood cells) in different industries where benzene is used was estimated on the basis of data from 24 985 factories in China. The prevalence was higher in factories in which benzene concentrations were high. A total of 2008 cases of leukopenia were found among 454 542 workers; the distribution of workers and cases and prevalences by industry are shown in Table 4. Twenty-four cases of aplastic anaemia and nine of leukaemia were found in the same investigation. Complete records were available for 17 of the cases of aplastic anaemia, and they were found to have been exposed to benzene for 3.5 months to 19 years. Most cases came from shoemaking and paint production factories, but a few were exposed during gluing and repairing and while packing insecticides. The benzene concentrations were generally greater than the hygienic standard of 40 mg/m^3, ranging from 93 to 1156 mg/m^3. The following example was cited: sandals were produced in a shoemaking factory, involving use of a 1:3 mixture of chlorobutadiene and benzene as an adhesive. Four cases of aplastic anaemia were detected among the 211 manual workers (1.9%) employed in this workshop during an eight-month period. All showed typical signs, symptoms and changes in blood and bone marrow and had been exposed to benzene for an average of 118.5 days at a daily mean concentration estimated to be about 1035.6 mg/m^3. The total amount of benzene inhaled was about 8278 g (Yin *et al.*, 1987; see p. 77).

Table 4. Prevalences of leukopenia among Chinese workers in industries where benzene is used

Industry	No. of workers	Cases	
		No.	%
Shoemaking	19 213	240	1.25
Paint production	12 359	67	0.54
Painting	101 379	415	0.41
Spray painting	175 313	682	0.39
Benzene refining	6 452	11	0.17
Chemical synthesis	42 766	190	0.44
Pharmaceuticals production	6 576	41	0.62
Rubber	13 877	56	0.40
Insulation varnish	24 378	101	0.41
Printing	15 453	56	0.30
Loading	870	7	0.80
Others	35 906	142	0.40
Total	454 542	2008	0.44

From Yin *et al.* (1987)

Cubatāo is a highly polluted industrial area of Brazil, near Sāo Paolo, where the main industries are steel and petrochemical works. Haematological analyses for steel workers from Cubatāo showed that 7.6% of them had fewer than 4000/mm^3 leukocytes and 12.1% had fewer than 2000/mm^3 neutrophils (de Almeida *et al.*, 1987). Another group of investigators conducted a morphological study of bone marrow from 95 neutropenic patients who were part of a population of 1000 workers who were removed from the working environment in Cubatāo because of haematological alterations. They were 20–60 years old and had presented with neutrophil counts lower than 2×10^9/L in repeated examinations. A characteristic cytological pattern was observed which was attributed by the authors to exposure to benzene; it consisted of a high prevalence of hypocellularity (77.9%), granulocytopenia (83.2%), megakaryocytopenia (65.3%), erythropenia, marrow eosinophilia, interstitial oedema and haemorrhagia in the stroma (Ruiz *et al.*, 1991).

Other health effects

A survey of workers in chromium electroplating plants in Brazil (Gomes, 1972) found that 86.8% of 303 workers in 94 plants in Sāo Paolo were affected by nasal lesions. Over one-third of the study population had ulcers of the nasal septum and approximately one-fourth showed septal perforations.

In China, nine cases with suspected or mild renal tubular damage were found among 65 workers exposed in a cadmium-refining plant (Liu *et al.*, 1985). The airborne concentrations of cadmium oxide ranged from 0.004 to 0.187 mg/m^3. The 5% prevalence of acro-osteolysis among workers in a vinyl chloride monomer production plant in Bogota, Colombia, was 10 times greater than the prevalence reported in US and Italian plants in the period before the standard was lowered (Michaels *et al.*, 1985).

A cross-sectional study was conducted of 107 South African foundry workers (Myers *et al.*, 1987). The prevalence of pneumoconiosis was 10.3% overall, increasing to 38% for workers with more than 15 years of service; dyspnoea was present in 38% of workers, chronic simple bronchitis in 15.9% and asthmatic symptoms in 27%.

References

de Almeida, T.V., Mendes, R., do Rego, J.C., Filho, D.C.M., Ribas, J.T. & Tonet, S.J. (1987) Haematological values in a group of workers in Cubatao. *Boletim*, **9**, 94–99 (in Portuguese)

Aragón, A., Pena, R. & Quintero, C. (1990) Lung disorders in a nationalized multinational gold mine, Mina El Limon, Nicaragua (Abstract). In: *Proceedings of the 23rd International Congress on Occupational Medicine, Montreal, Canada, 22–28 September 1990*, p. 242

Ballal, S.G. (1986) Respiratory symptoms and occupational bronchitis in chromite ore miners, Sudan. *J. Trop. Med. Hyg.*, **89**, 223–228

Baloyi, R. (1989) *Exposure to Asbestos among Chrysotile Miners, Millers and Mine Residents and Asbestosis in Zimbabwe*, Helsinki, Institute of Occupational Health

Chen, S.Y., Hayes, R.B., Liang, S.R., Li, Q.G., Stewart, P.A. & Blair, A. (1990) Mortality experience of haematite mine workers in China. *Br. J. Ind. Med.*, **47**, 175–181

Chia, S.-E., Chia, K.-S., Phoon, W.-H. & Lee, H.-P. (1991) Silicosis and lung cancer among Chinese granite workers. *Scand. J. Work Environ. Health*, **17**, 170–174

Christiani, D.C. & Gu, X.-Q. (1988) The People's Republic of China. In: Levy, B. & Wegman, D., eds, *Occupational Health. Recognizing and Preventing Work Related Disease*, Boston, Little, Brown, pp. 560–568

Colombian Government (1987) Decree No. 778 of 30 April 1987 amending the list of occupational diseases contained in Section 201 of the Basic Labour Code. *Diaro Of.*, 37868, 11–12 (in Spanish)

Cook, W.A., ed. (1987) *Occupational Exposure Limits—Worldwide*, Washington DC, American Industrial Hygiene Association

Cullen, M.R. & Baloyi, R.S. (1990) Prevalence of pneumoconiosis among coal and heavy metal miners in Zimbabwe. *Am. J. Ind. Med.*, **17**, 677–682

Cullen, M.R. & Baloyi, R.S. (1991) Chrysotile asbestos and health in Zimbabwe: I. Analysis of miners and millers compensated for asbestos-related diseases since independence (1980). *Am. J. Ind. Med.*, **19**, 161–169

Cullen, M.R., Lopez-Carrillo, L., Alli, B., Pace, P.E., Shalat, S.L. & Baloyi, R.S. (1991) Chrysotile asbestos and health in Zimbabwe: II. Health status survey of active miners and millers. *Am. J. Ind. Med.*, **19**, 171–182

Ehrlich, R.I., Rees, D. & Zwi, A.B. (1988) Silicosis in non-mining industry on the Witwatersrand. *S. Afr. Med. J.*, **73**, 704–708

El Batawi, M.A. (1986) The third Theodore F. Hatch symposium lecture. *Ann. Am. Conf. Gov. Ind. Hyg.*, **14**, 3–15

Fatma, N., Jain, A.K. & Rahman, Q. (1991) Frequency of sister chromatid exchange and chromosomal aberrations in asbestos cement workers. *Br. J. Ind. Med.*, **48**, 103–105

Goldsmith, J.R. (1985) Occupational health in Chinese metallurgical industries: report based on a visit. *Am. J. Ind. Med.*, **7**, 353–357

Gomes, E.R. (1972) Incidence of chromium-induced lesions among electroplating workers in Brazil. *Ind. Med.*, **41**, 21–25

Government of Hong Kong (1987) The Employees Compensation Ordinance (Amendment of Section Schedule) Order 1987. L.N. 52 of 1987. Dated 17 February 1987. *Hong Kong Government Gazette*, **129** (Legal Suppl. No. 2 to No. 9), B140–B141

Gu, X.-Q. (1985) The role of early detection in the prevention of occupational disease — a review of work in the People's Republic of China. *Scand. J. Work Environ. Health*, **11** (Suppl. 4), 7–9

Gupta, S.P., Bajaj, A., Jain, A.L. & Vasudeva, Y.L. (1972) Clinical and radiological studies in silicosis: based on a study of the disease amongst stone-cutters. *Indian J. Med. Res.*, **60**, 1309–1315

IARC (1987) *IARC Monographs on the Evaluation of the Carcinogenic Risk of Chemicals to Humans*, Vol. 42, *Silica and Some Silicates*, Lyon

ILO (1984) *Securité dans l'Utilisation de l'Amiante* [Safety in the Use of Asbestos], Geneva

Irwig, L.M., du Toit, R.S.J., Sluis-Cremer, G.K., Solomon, A., Glyn Thomas, R.G., Hamel, P.P.H., Webster, I. & Hastie, T. (1979) Risk of asbestosis in crocidolite and amosite mines in South Africa. *Ann. N.Y. Acad. Sci.*, **330**, 35–52

Kurppa, K., Sakari, W.D.O., Wambugu, A.W., Mubisi, A.S., Rantanen, J. & Tuppurainen, M. (1984) Research on occupational health problems in Kenyan industries: diseases caused by calcined diatomite, asbestos, cotton, and lead. In: Tuppurainen, M. & Kurppa, K., eds, *Proceedings of the First ILO–Finnish–Tanzanian Symposium on Occupational Health, 8–10 October, Marangu, Moshi, Tanzania*, Geneva, ILO, pp. 76–79

Liu, Y.-Z., Huang, J.-X., Luo, C.-M., Xu, B.-H. & Zhang, C.-J. (1985) Effects of cadmium on cadmium smelter workers. *Scand. J. Work Environ. Health*, **11** (Suppl. 4), 29–32

McDermott, M., Bevan, M.M., Elmes, P.C., Allardice, J.T. & Bradley, A.C. (1982) Lung function and radiographic change in chrysotile workers in Swaziland. *Br. J. Ind. Med.*, **39**, 338–343

Michaels, D., Barrera, C. & Gacharná, M.G. (1985) Economic development and occupational health in Latin America: new directions for public health in less developed countries. *Am. J. Public Health*, **75**, 536–542

Mohamed, I.Y. (1990) Asbestos–cement pneumoconiosis: first surgically confirmed case in Kuwait. *Am. J. Ind. Med.*, **17**, 241–245

Myers, J. (1981) The social context of occupational disease: asbestos and South Africa. *Int. J. Health Serv.*, **11**, 227–245

Myers, J.E., Garisch, D., Myers, H.S., Cornell, J.E. & Rwexu, R.D. (1985) A respiratory epidemiological study of stevedores intermittently exposed to asbestos in a South African port. *Am. J. Ind. Med.*, **7**, 273–283

Myers, J.E., Garisch, D., Myers, H.S. & Cornell, J.E. (1987) A respiratory epidemiological survey of workers in a small South African foundry. *Am. J. Ind. Med.*, **12**, 1–9

Ng, T.P. (1986) A case–referent study of cancer of the nasal cavity and sinuses in Hong Kong. *Int. J. Epidemiol.*, **15**, 171–175

Ng, T.P. (1992) Occupational lung disease — mineral dusts. In: Jeyaratnam, J., ed., *Occupational Health in Developing Countries*, Oxford, Oxford University Press, pp. 287–303

Ng, T.P. & O'Kelly, F.J. (1987) Silicosis prevalence in granite quarry and contruction workers in Hong Kong. *J. Hong Kong Med. Assoc.*, **39**, 160–162

Ng, T.P., Phoon, W.H., Lee, H.S., Ng, Y.L. & Tan, K.T. (1992) An epidemiological survey of respiratory morbidity among granite quarry workers in Singapore: radiological abnormalities. *Ann. Acad. Med. Singapore*, **21**, 305–311

Nogueira, D.P., Certain, D., Brólio, R., Garrafa, N.M. & Shibata, H. (1981) Silicosis among workers in the ceramic industry in Jundiai, SP (Brazil). *Rev. Saude Publ.*, **15**, 263–271 (in Portuguese)

Noweir, M.H. (1986) Occupational health in developing countries with special reference to Egypt. *Am. J. Ind. Med.*, **9**, 125–141

Ogaram, D.A. (1990) Potential hazards in Uganda. *Afr. Newslett. Occup. Health Saf.*, **31 August**, 10–11

Packard, R.M. (1989) Industrial production, health and disease in sub-Saharan Africa. *Soc. Sci. Med.*, **28**, 475–496

Pinell, L.F. (1976) Frequency of silicosis and silico-tuberculosis among mine workers in Bolivia: an epidemiological study. *Bull. Int. Union Against TB*, **51**, 577–582

Prenafeta, J. (1984) Pneumoconiosis in Chile. *Rev. Méd. Chile*, **112**, 511–515 (in Spanish)

Rees, D. & Kielkowski, D. (1991) Dust and pneumoconiosis in the South African ceramic industry. *S. Afr. J. Sci.*, **87**, 493–495

Ruiz, M.A., Vassallo, J. & De Souca, C.A. (1991) Morphologic study of the bone marrow of neutropenic patients exposed to benzene in the metallurgical industry of Cubatão, São Paulo, Brazil (Letter). *J. Occup. Med.*, **33**, 83

Saiyed, H.N., Parikh, D.J., Ghodasara, N.B., Sharma, Y.K., Patel, G.C., Chatterjee, S.K. & Chatterjee, B.B. (1985) Silicosis in slate pencil workers: I. An environmental and medical study. *Am. J. Ind. Med.*, **8**, 127–133

Sakari, W.D.O. (1990) Occupational lung disorders due to mineral dust in Kenya. *East Afr. Newslett. Occup. Health Saf.*, **31 August**, 6–7

Scansetti, G., Coscia, G.C., Pisani, W. & Rubino, G.F. (1975) Cement, asbestos, and cement–asbestos pneumonoconioses. *Arch. Environ. Health.*, **30**, 272–275

Singh, A. (1977) The prevalence of silicosis among granite quarry workers, of the government sector, in Peninsular Malaysia. *Med. J. Malaysia*, **31**, 277–280

Solomons, K. (1984) Malignant mesothelioma—clinical and epidemiological features. A report of 80 cases. *S. Afr. Med. J.*, **66**, 407–412

Uragoda, S.G. (1989) Graphite pneumoconiosis and its declining prevalence in Sri Lanka. *J. Trop. Med. Hyg.*, **92**, 422–424

Uragoda, C.G., Sheriffdeen, A.H. & Amerasinghe, A. (1983) A case of asbestos associated disease in Sri Lanka. *Ceylon Med. J.*, **28**, 247–249

White, N.W., Chetty, R. & Bateman, E.D. (1991) Silicosis among gemstone workers in South Africa: tiger's-eye pneumoconiosis. *Am. J. Ind. Med.*, **19**, 205–213

Yin, S.N., Li, Q., Liu, Y., Tian, F., Du, C. & Jin, C. (1987) Occupational exposure to benzene in China. *Br. J. Ind. Med.*, **44**, 192–195

Part IV

Primary Prevention and Control

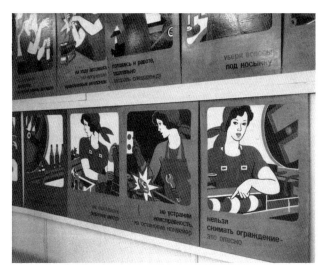

Above: Education is essential in the prevention and control of occupational hazards. These safety information boards in a Russian textile factory improve the workers' awareness of risks.

Photo by J. Maillard, courtesy of International Labour Office

Below: Personal protection can often help to reduce exposure, but may be costly and inappropriate for use in hot, humid climates.

Photo: Courtesy of World Health Organization and Ministère des forêts du Québec.

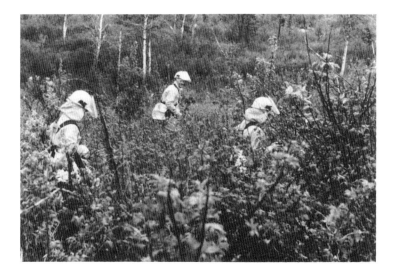

Chapter 9. International and National Measures for Prevention and Control

This chapter comprises reviews of the work of the two United Nations organizations that have a direct interest in the prevention of occupational cancer: WHO and ILO. It also presents the findings of the IARC survey on national legislation on chemicals recognized as carcinogens and on occupational diseases recognized as being caused by chemical carcinogens.

Action of WHO (M.I. Mikheev)

Cancer of occupational origin is one facet of the WHO Workers' Health Programme and of other, related programmes, such as those on cancer, the prevention of environmental pollution and health education. At the First World Health Assembly in 1948, WHO ranked the study of cancer number six in priority (WHA1.5). In 1957, the World Health Assembly requested the Director-General 'to include in the epidemiological work on cancer due reference to occupational and other environmental conditions likely to have an influence on the frequency of the various forms of the disease and therefore an etiological significance'. In 1959, a Scientific Group on Cancer Research formulated a comprehensive cancer programme, with the recommendation to 'promote international efforts in the study of industrial and occupational cancer'. Two activities were seen as essential: promotion of the identification of carcinogens by improving the accuracy of employment and medical records in occupations in which the presence of carcinogens is suspected; and the establishment of registers of cancer patients for whom the disease is alleged to be associated with specific causative factors not already established as carcinogens.

The Twenty-sixth World Health Assembly considered '... that the main effort in cancer research should be made by the national research organizations of Member States, but that their activities should be coordinated ...' and '... that they would cover, inter alia, the standardization of methods and of terminology, epidemiological studies, and the development of methods for the early diagnosis and treatment of cancer and of preventive measures, including the identification and removal of carcinogens from the environment' (WHA26.61).

The WHO Cancer Control Programme is based on the concept that enough knowledge now exists about cancer for effective action to be taken that will significantly reduce cancer morbidity and mortality worldwide, if implemented properly. The corresponding World Health Assembly Resolution (WHA35.30) urged Member States to strengthen or—where lacking—to consider initiating the development of cancer control measures as an integral part of national health plans. As emphasized in the Eighth General Programme of Work covering the period

1990–95 (WHO, 1987), prevention is a priority among cancer control activities, as most cases of cancer of the lung, oral cavity and liver, as well as some other common forms of cancer, can be prevented. WHO has emphasized the prevention of cancer through healthy life-styles and will foster national health education to this effect (WHO/EURO, 1991; Rothwell, 1992).

The WHO Workers' Health Programme has received strong support and specific guidance from a number of resolutions of the World Health Assembly, the Executive Board and Regional Committees. Even at the First World Health Assembly in 1948, the subject of industrial hygiene was ranked number two in priority within the topic 'Public Health Administration' (WHA1.51). WHO activities in the area of occupational cancer have taken many directions, including the formulation of standards and promotion of coordinated activities for strengthening the legal, administrative and occupational frameworks necessary to ensure health and safety in workplaces.

WHO promotes the development and publication of methods for the early detection of health impairment of workers (WHO, 1986). Criteria have been formalized for diagnosing occupational diseases caused by chemical and physical factors, many of which are also carcinogenic. Detection of health impairment at early stages or before cancer development is an important approach in occupational cancer control. An efficient early detection system depends on certain conditions: appropriate regulations must exist for identification of health hazards; appropriate occupational health services must exist to organize and carry out health examinations; and adequate methods for health examination must be available.

Control of occupational cancer involves several types of activity. Carcinogens in the occupational environment must be identified, and occupational exposure of workers to those carcinogens should be eliminated, predominantly by technical measures, when and where possible. Unfortunately, the present levels of technology and of national economies do not permit the exclusion of all occupational exposures to carcinogens; therefore, the concept that exposure should be as low as possible has been promoted. As the carcinogenic transformation of cells is still not well understood, so-called technical exposure limits are set in some countries for the control of many carcinogenic substances (Commission for the Investigation of Health Hazards and Chemical Compounds in the Work Area, 1991). Such limits can be a useful stimulus for developing new control methods which, in turn, may lead to further lowering of the threshold limit values and thus lowering workers' exposures.

The series of *IARC Monographs on the Evaluation of Carcinogenic Risks to Humans* (see Chapter 4) have been of major significance in the identification of occupational carcinogens. The critical analyses of data in the *Monographs* are intended to assist national and international authorities in formulating policies and decisions concerning preventive measures, and to define those areas in which additional research is needed.

The identification of carcinogenic industrial chemicals and processes initiates a series of preventive and control measures, including replacement of carcinogenic agents by noncarcinogenic or less harmful agents. When complete elimination is impossible, the number of workers exposed to them and the duration and degree of such exposure should be reduced to the greatest possible extent, at least to a minimum that is compatible with safety. These principles, as well as the concept of hazard communication, which requires that workers be provided with all available information on the dangers involved and the preventive measures to be taken (including information on medical examinations or other tests or investigations that are necessary to evaluate their exposure and supervise their state of health in relation to the occupational hazard), have been promoted by WHO in close collaboration with ILO and other international organizations (ILO, 1974; WHO/EURO, 1990).

Since 1976, the WHO Office of Occupational Health has developed internationally recommended health-based occupational exposure limits. Documents on metals (cadmium, lead, manganese, mercury), solvents (toluene, xylene, carbon disulfide, trichloroethylene) and pesticides (carbaryl, malathion, lindane, dinitro-*ortho*-cresol) have been published in the WHO Technical Report Series (WHO, 1980, 1981, 1982). The aim of the project is to provide decision-makers and their experts with data on the relationship between level of exposure and health effects, on which to base decisions on operational occupational exposure limits.

In the early 1980s, WHO formulated a new global strategy in order to achieve the target of 'Health for All by the Year 2000'. In Resolution WHO30.43, it is proclaimed that '... the attainment by all the peoples of the world by the year 2000 of a level of health that will permit them to lead a socially and economically productive life is the main target of governments and of WHO.' If we are to meet this target, the prevention and control of occupational hazards, and especially carcinogens, must be improved considerably.

In developing countries, which lack the economic means and health services, several circumstances limit the efficiency of preventive measures in occupational health. These include:

(i)   obsolete workers' health legislation and, in particular, a total absence of specific legislation on prevention of occupational cancer in most countries;

(ii)   the absence of 'threshold limit values' for occupational exposures to hazardous substances;

(iii)   shortage of qualified occupational health manpower, particularly occupational hygienists, and, consequently, the absence of either regular environmental monitoring of workplaces or periodic monitoring of health;

(iv)   the absence of or poor notification of occupational diseases;

(v)   a paucity of epidemiological studies on the relationship between occupational stress and health impairment;

(vi)   the low average level of engineering controls in most industries and particularly in small-scale industries; and

(vii)   lack of specific training in occupational health of staff in enforcing agencies, such as labour and factory inspectorates.

Workers' health education plays a crucial role in the control of risks for occupational cancer: all of the above-mentioned legislative, technological and environmental control measures may be applied, but they will not be sufficiently effective unless accompanied by self-protection. Existing knowledge on occupational cancer prevention has not been implemented fully in developing countries, but they must have access to the experience gained in countries with advanced technology. International organizations can serve to transfer such information, not only to medical officers but also to engineers, chemists, administrators and workers on the factory floor.

Small-scale industries in developing countries represent a particular problem, as awareness of carcinogenic hazards is inevitably more limited than in large-scale organizations. The provision of specific education and information to personnel employed in small-scale industries is thus of considerable importance.

Appropriate measures to prevent cancer in the workplace can form the basis for international cooperation in the field of occupational cancer, as stated in the Report to the Twenty-seventh World Health Assembly, through:

(i)   the development and standardization of methods for the detection, identification and measurement of occupational carcinogenic agents;

(ii)   the identification and characterization of groups at high risk for cancer because of occupational and/or associated community exposure to carcinogens;

(iii)   the development, application and evaluation of methods for protection against known occupational carcinogenic agents;

(iv)   the development of data resources for investigating cancer risk, especially through population-based cancer registries;

(v)   the development of screening and diagnostic techniques for early detection of occupational cancer;

(vi)   the delivery of preventive health care through occupational services and, when not feasible, through general health services, using the primary health care approach;

(vii)   the proper education and training of staff of health services in the prevention and control of occupational cancer; and

(viii) the education and training of administrators, employers, supervisors and workers with regard to health hazards and their prevention and to active participation in occupational cancer control.

Efficient control and prevention of occupational cancer require the development of comprehensive, multidisciplinary national programmes on occupational health, which can undertake practical tasks such as problem assessment, planning for action, implementation and evaluation. In countries where comprehensive occupational health services cannot be organized for all workers, action should be taken to provide the essential core of such services to those workers who are in greatest need. Core services, as defined by EUR/ICP/OCU, comprise identification of hazards at the workplace and assessment of their health consequences, placing of workers in jobs compatible with their health status, surveillance and follow-up of the health status of workers exposed to hazardous agents at work, provision for diagnosis and, when appropriate, treatment of occupational diseases. They should also include assessment of exposure to carcinogenic agents, by monitoring in the working environment and biological monitoring and health surveillance of exposed workers.

Action and guidelines of ILO (K. Kurppa and J. Takala)

Background

The ILO was founded after the Versailles Peace Treaty in 1919 as a response to the call for social justice in international relations. The main idea was to promote social progress by means of international agreements, without distorting competition between countries. ILO's mandate is to ensure respect of workers' fundamental rights worldwide, to attempt to achieve full employment, better living standards, fair distribution of rewards of progress and protection of life and health of the workers, and to support cooperation between employers and workers in all fields of common interest. Protection of workers against sickness, disease and injury arising out of their employment by improving conditions of labour was thus one of the main reasons for the foundation of the ILO. In 1946, it became the first specialized agency of the United Nations and now cooperates closely with other specialized agencies within the system, such as WHO.

ILO is based on the International Labour Conference, which is a general assembly held in June every year, and it has a governing body and a permanent secretariat, the International Labour Office, which is based in Geneva. Tripartism is the distinguishing feature of ILO: governments, employers and workers are equally represented, and all decisions are made after discussion and negotiation in a tripartite assembly. ILO also works through subsidiary bodies, such as regional conferences, industrial committees and panels of experts.

ILO activities fall into three major categories: setting of standards, research and dissemination of information, and technical cooperation. In matters of occupational safety and health, the activities are typically designed to back up national action: ILO Conventions and Recommendations are used when drafting national legislation; model codes and codes of practice assist in designing national regulations; manuals, guides and technical publications support national activities in technical and medical inspection; publications, seminars, courses, congresses, symposia and fellowships provide appropriate information to administrators, employers and workers; and technical cooperation covers the operational assistance of ILO to progress in social and labour issues in the Member States.

Several ILO activities aim specifically at the prevention of occupational cancer. Direct examples are the adoption and promotion of the Occupational Cancer Convention and Recommendation (ILO, 1974) and publication of a book on prevention and control of occupational cancer (ILO, 1988). Separate ILO programmes deal with certain important chemical and physical carcinogens, such as ionizing radiation, asbestos and benzene. Many other programmes address the problem in more indirect ways, through general improvement of working conditions and the environment and rectification of the associated juridical area.

Standards

A fundamental task of the Organisation is to set standards. ILO standards consist of conventions and recommendations (Table 1). When a country ratifies a convention, it becomes a binding legal obligation, and its provisions must by adopted by national legislation. Recommendations are not legally binding documents, but they can be used as guides when writing national regulations. The countries that ratify a convention are obliged to establish appropriate administrative structures to supervise its implementation. In consultation with the most representative organizations of employers and workers concerned, the government must specify the persons or bodies with whom the obligation rests to comply with the provisions of the convention. The government also provides the necessary inspection services for supervising application of the convention.

Table 1. ILO conventions and recommendations of importance to the prevention of occupational cancer

Convention or recommendation	Date
Radiation Protection Convention No. 115	1960
Radiation Protection Recommendation No. 114	1960
Benzene Convention No. 136	1971
Benzene Recommendation No. 144	1971
Occupational Cancer Convention No. 139	1974
Occupational Cancer Recommendation No. 147	1974
Working Environment Convention No. 148	1977
Working Environment Recommendation No. 156	1977
Occupational Health Services Convention No. 161	1985
Occupational Health Services Recommendation No. 171	1985
Asbestos Convention No. 162	1986
Asbestos Recommendation No. 172	1986
Chemicals Convention No. 170	1990
Chemicals Recommendation No. 177	1990

The International Labour Conference discussed the prevention of occupational cancer and protection of workers against carcinogens in 1973 and 1974, and the Occupational Cancer Convention concerning prevention and control of occupational hazards caused by carcinogenic substances and agents was adopted in 1974. That Convention specifies the principles to be adopted by countries for the prevention of occupational cancer. A leading principle is that every effort be made to replace carcinogenic substances and agents to which workers may be exposed by noncarcinogenic substances or agents. It also states that the number of workers exposed to carcinogenic substances or agents and the duration and degree of such exposure should be reduced to the minimum compatible with safety. Workers must be provided with such medical examinations or biological or other tests or investigations during the period of employment and thereafter as are necessary to evalute their exposure and supervise their state of health. By 1992, the following Member States had ratified the Occupational Cancer Convention: Afghanistan, Argentina, Brazil, the former Czechoslovakia, Denmark, Ecuador, Egypt, Finland, Germany, Guinea, Guyana, Hungary, Iceland, Iraq, Italy, Japan, Nicaragua, Norway, Peru, Sweden, Switzerland, the Syrian Arab Republic, Uruguay, Venezuala and the former Yugoslavia.

The Occupational Cancer Recommendation (see Table 1) gives more detailed guidance concerning prevention and control of occupational hazards due to carcinogenic agents. The general provisions of the Recommendation suggest that employers make every effort to use work processes that do not involve the formation and emission into the working environment of carcinogens as main products, intermediates, by-products, waste products and others. If complete elimination of a carcinogen is not possible, employers are to use all appropriate measures, in consultation with workers and their organizations, to eliminate exposures or reduce them to a minimum in terms of numbers exposed, duration of exposure and degree of exposure. Employers are to make arrangements for the systematic surveillance of the duration and degree of exposure to carcinogens in the working environment.

Preventive measures include periodic determination by competent authorities of carcinogenic substances and agents to which occupational exposure should be prohibited or made subject to authorization or control. Information and education needs are to be fulfilled by the competent authority, by drawing up suitable educational guides for both employers and workers on carcinogenic substances and agents. Employers are to ensure that appropriate indications are available to any worker at the workplace about carcinogenic hazards and that workers are properly instructed before assignment and regularly thereafter.

Publications

The ILO publication *Occupational Cancer: Prevention and Control* is a valuable collection of materials useful to both occupational health and safety administrators and professionals at the workplace. The first edition in 1977 provided guidance to those responsible for applying the principles of the Occupational Cancer Convention and Recommendation. An updated edition of the book (ILO, 1988) was issued with the technical help of IARC, in which the text was completely revised and expanded in the light of new knowledge.

The book describes the basic principles of the necessary technical measures and of substitution, special studies to minimize the duration of dangerous operations, design of installations, operating instructions, personal protective measures and emergencies. It also describes workplace and biological monitoring to prevent undue exposure to carcinogens, health surveillance and the establishment of registers. Problems in establishing occupational standards for carcinogens are described, and the classification of carcinogens for the purpose of legislation is discussed. Carcinogenic chemicals, physical agents and processes listed by the ILO Panel of Consultants on Occupational Cancer are given, and appendices include lists of carcinogenic agents and industrial processes identified in the *IARC Monographs* and several national lists of carcinogenic substances.

The *Encyclopaedia on Occupational Health and Safety* is a collection of practically orientated information. After more than a decade of preparation, the third version, a two-volume reference work of 2400 pages, was published in 1983 (ILO, 1983); it includes articles written by international specialists. The fourth edition will be published in 1995, not only as a hard copy publication but also on a CD-ROM disc.

The preface to the third edition defines the target groups as follows:

> The encyclopaedia is intended for all those who have administrative or moral responsibilities for safeguarding workers' health and safety, especially in developing countries, and for all those who have technical responsibilities in this field but do not have at their disposal adequate library facilities or international selections of recent documents on the many and vast fields covered by, or related to, occupational health and safety.

The *Encyclopaedia* provides industrial physicians, nurses, hygienists, ergonomists and safety specialists with a compendium of practical knowledge in their field and familiarizes them with the technical features of prevention. It also informs engineers and technicians about the biological and social aspects of their work and makes knowledge about occupational safety and health accessible to employers and trade union representatives. Articles on occupational cancer and on environmental cancer and related issues are supplemented by specific articles on several carcinogenic chemicals and physical agents, such as benzene, asbestos, chromium and ionizing radiation. Each article includes recommendations for preventive measures.

Full-text data base

Prevention of occupational cancer is one of the targets of a recently initiated ILO technical cooperation programme, the Asian−Pacific Regional Programme on Occupational Safety and Health (ASIA-OSH), which covers 21 countries or areas in Asia and the Pacific. The programme is funded by the Finnish Development Aid Agency. ASIA-OSH is a sister project for a similar long-term ILO programme, also funded by the Finnish Agency, in 20 English-speaking African countries, which has been operational for more than two years, with the object of occupational safety and health training and dissemination of information.

Computers can improve access to information, and one approach is to develop databases tailored to local purposes, distributed on discs or by electronic communication and stored on hard or floppy discs. Advantages include low cost and flexibility; the procedure also offers the possibility of combining international information with local experience. A database providing guidance for the prevention of occupational cancer is being prepared within the ASIA-OSH programme. It will include full-text information about the ILO Convention and Recommendation concerning prevention and control of exposure to carcinogenic substances and agents, other relevant conventions and recommendations, extracts from the ILO book on occupational cancer, international and national lists of carcinogenic substances and agents, articles about occupational cancer from the ILO *Encyclopaedia*, guidance on dealing with carcinogens and other practical material. The strategy is to repackage information from the United Nations, other agencies and selected government sources into practical collections of knowledge and models.

The ASIA-OSH programme also produces databases on important agents, such as benzene and asbestos. The diskettes will contain the appropriate ILO instruments, a model standard if available, guidelines and safety sheets, guidelines for hygienic methods and medical surveillance, precautions against carcinogenicity, dealing with emergencies, disposal, treatment of spills and leaks, first aid and other practical items. The work is shared by experts from the participating Asian and Pacific countries. The databases are disseminated throughout the Region by the CIS Centre network and by national counterparts.

The multilayer structure of the ASIA-OSH databases will allow the development of national and local information systems on hazardous substances by national and local experts in the same database. The internationally collected information thus serves as a background and model, which can be modified according to cultural and geographical realities.

National control measures (E. Matos and C. Partensky)

In preparation for this publication, a survey was carried out at IARC on national legislation on chemicals recognized as carcinogens and on occupational diseases recognized as being caused by chemical carcinogens. The methods used and detailed results are given in the Appendix.

Legislation on chemicals recognized as carcinogens

Table 2 presents the information on chemicals included in national lists of countries in Latin America, Asia and the Middle East as carcinogens or potential carcinogens. The Table is not comprehensive, but it provides relevant examples of current practices.

The Table was constructed from responses to the IARC survey, from *Occupational Exposure Limits—Worldwide* by W.A. Cook (1987), which includes information from the American Conference of Governmental Industrial Hygienists (ACGIH) for 1984–85, references obtained through bibliographical searches, material sent by WHO (HLE Unit) and ILO (CIS) and personal communications. In some regions (e.g. Chile and Hong Kong), the lists of substances to be prohibited or controlled make no mention of carcinogenicity. In other cases, occupational exposure limits, which are usually time-weighted average concentrations, are included in general lists of hazardous or dangerous substances, although such limits are often not based only on health considerations and may not be enforced in practice. The tables include the IARC classifications up to 1993 (IARC, 1993) and the 1991–92 list of ACGIH (1991).

Most developing countries follow the classifications and exposure limits given by the ACGIH; their legislation also states that they will accept any updated reviews of the values. For example, in Colombia and Ecuador, the limit values for carcinogens are identical to the ACGIH threshold limit values, whereas minor differences are found in Argentina, Brazil and Mexico (Cook, 1987, 1989). Specific regulations on carcinogens are as follows:

Argentina: The regulation of carcinogens is only slightly different from that of the ACGIH (Cook, 1987). A regulation from the National Direction of Occupational Safety and Health modified a Disposition of 1989 listing carcinogenic substances and agents and established a registry of the enterprises that produce, import, use or obtain as

Table 2. Agents included in national lists as carcinogens or possible carcinogens and time-weighted averages

Agent	IARC (1993)	ACGIH (1991–92)	Latin America						
			Argentina	Brazil	Chile	Cuba	Mexico	Peru	Venezuela
Acrylonitrile	2A	A2 2 ppm (4.3 mg/m3) (S)	2 ppm (S) (P)	16 ppm (S)	1.6 ppm (P)	10 mg/m3	2 ppm (S) (P)		2 ppm (4.5 mg/m3)
4-Aminobiphenyl	1	A1 (S)							x
Aniline	3	2 ppm (7.6 mg/m3) (S)	2 ppm (S)	4 ppm	1.6 ppm (S)		2 ppm (S)		5 ppm (S)
Antimony trioxide production	2B	A2 0.5 mg/m3 (compound)					1 mg/m3		x
Arsenic and compounds (As)	1	0.2 mg/m3 (soluble compound)	0.2 mg/m3		0.16 mg/m3	0.6 mg/m3	0.2 mg/m3	0.5 mg/m3	0.5 mg/m3
Arsenic trioxide production (As)	1	A2					0.5 mg/m3		x
Asbestos (all forms)	1	A1 0.2–2 f/cm3[a]	0.2–2 f/cm3	2 f/cm3	0.2–1.6 f/cm3	1 f/cm3	2 f/cm3		0.5 f/cm3 >5 μm
Asphalt fumes	3	5 mg/m3	5 mg/m3		4 mg/m3		5 mg/m3		5 mg/m3
Benzene (Benzol)	1	A2 10 ppm (32 mg/m3)[b]	10 ppm	8 ppm	8 ppm (S)		10 ppm	25 ppm	10 ppm
Benzidine and its salts	1	A1 (S)	(P) (S)		(P)		(P)		x
Benzyl chloride	2B	1 ppm (5.2 mg/m3)	1 ppm				1 ppm		1 ppm
Beryllium and compounds (Be)	1	A2 0.002 mg/m3	0.002 mg/m3				0.002 mg/m3	0.005 mg/m3	0.002 mg/m3
Bis(chloromethyl)ether	1	A1 0.001 ppm (0.0047 mg/m3)	0.001 ppm		0.0008 ppm				0.001 ppm
1,3-Butadiene	2A	A2 10 ppm (22 mg/m3)	10 ppm	780 ppm			1000 ppm		1000 ppm
Cadmium and compounds (Cd)	1	0.05 mg/m3[c]	0.05 mg/m3						0.05 mg/m3
Cadmium oxide, production (Cd)	1	0.05 mg/m3[c]	0.05 mg/m3			0.1 mg/m3			
Carbon tetrachloride	2B	A2 5 ppm (31 mg/m3) (S)	5 ppm (S)	8 ppm	4 ppm (S)		10 ppm (S)		5 ppm
Chloroform	2B	A2 10 ppm (49 mg/m3)	10 ppm	20 ppm	8 ppm		5 ppm		10 ppm
Chloromethyl methyl ether	1	A2			(P)				x
Chromate lead (Pb) (Cr)	1	A2 0.05 mg/m3 (0.012 mg/m3)	0.05 mg/m3	x			0.05 mg/m3		0.05 mg/m3
Chromate zinc (Cr)	1	A1 0.01 mg/m3	0.01 mg/m3						0.05 mg/m3
Chromic acid (dichromic) and salts (Cr)	1	0.05 mg/m3	x						
Chromite ore processing (Cr)		A1 0.05 mg/m3	0.05 mg/m3				0.05 mg/m3		0.05 mg/m3
Chromium[VI] compounds (Cr)	1	A1 0.05 mg/m3	0.05 mg/m3				0.5 mg/m3		0.05 mg/m3
Chromium and compounds (Cr)		0.05–0.5 mg/m3	0.05 mg/m3	x	0.04 mg/m3	1.0 mg/m3	0.5 mg/m3	0.5 mg/m3	0.1 mg/m3
Chrysene	3	A2							x
Coal-tar pitch (volatile, soluble in benzene)	1	A2 0.2 mg/m3 (0.012 mg/m3)	0.2 mg/m3		4 mg/m3		0.2 mg/m3		x
para-Dichlorobenzene	2B	75 ppm (451 mg/m3)[d]	75 ppm				75 ppm		75 ppm
3,3'-Dichlorobenzidine	2B	A2 (S)							x
Dimethylcarbamoyl chloride	2A	A2							x
1,1-Dimethylhydrazine	2B	A2 0.5 ppm (1.2 mg/m3)[e] (S)	0.5 ppm (S)	0.4 ppm (S)			0.6 ppm		0.5 ppm (S)
Dimethylsulfate	2A	A2 0.1 ppm (0.52 mg/m3) (S)	0.8 ppm	0.4 mg/m3 (S)	0.08 ppm (S)		0.1 ppm (S)		0.1 ppm (S)
Diphenylamine		10 mg/m3	10 mg/m3				10 mg/m3		10 mg/m3

Table 2 (contd)

Agent	IARC (1993)	ACGIH (1991–92)	Latin America						
			Argentina	Brazil	Chile	Cuba	Mexico	Peru	Venezuela
Ethylene dibromide	2A	A2 (S)	(S)		(P)		26 ppm (S)		20 ppm (S)
Ethyleneimine		0.5 ppm (0.88 mg/m^3) (S)	0.5 ppm (S)	0.4 ppm (S)			0.5 ppm (S)		0.5 ppm (S)
Ethylene oxide	2A	A2 1 ppm (1.8 mg/m^3)	1 ppm	39 ppm	8 ppm		45 ppm		1 ppm
Formaldehyde	2A	A2 1 ppm (1.2 mg/m^3)[f]	1 ppm	1.6 ppm	1.6 ppm	0.8 ppm	2 ppm		1 ppm
Hexachloro-1,3-butadiene	3	A2 0.02 ppm (0.21 mg/m^3) (S)	0.02 ppm						0.02 ppm
Hexamethylphosphoramide	2B	A2 (S)	(S)						x
Hydrazine	2B	A2 0.1 ppm (0.13 mg/m^3)[g] (S)	0.1 ppm	0.08 ppm (S)		0.1 ppm	0.1 ppm (S)		0.1 ppm (S)
Lead	2B	0.15 mg/m^3	0.15 mg/m^3	0.1 mg/m^3	0.12 mg/m^3		0.15 mg/m^3		0.15 mg/m^3
Methyl iodide	3	A2 2 ppm (12 mg/m^3) (S)	2 ppm				5 ppm (S)		2 ppm (S)
4,4'-Methylene bis(2-chloroaniline) (MOCA)	2A	A2 0.02 ppm (0.22 mg/m^3)[h] (S)	0.02 ppm				0.02 ppm (S)	0.02 ppm (S)	
Methylene chloride	2B	A2 50 ppm (174 mg/m^3)	50 ppm	156 ppm			100 ppm		200 ppm
Methylhydrazine		A2 0.2 ppm (0.38 mg/m^3)[i] (S)	0.2 ppm	0.16 ppm (S/C)		0.2 ppm (S)	0.2 ppm (S)	0.2 ppm (S)	
2-Naphthylamine	1	A1	(P)		(P)		x		x
Nickel carbonyl (Ni)	1	0.05 ppm (0.12 mg/m^3)[i]	0–10 mg/m^3	0.28 mg/m^3			0.35 mg/m^3		0.35 mg/m^3
Nickel sulfide (roast, fume, dust) (Ni)	1	A1 1 mg/m^3[i]	1 mg/m^3				1 mg/m^3		1 mg/m^3
Nickel compounds (Ni)	1	0.1–1 mg/m^3[i]	0.1 mg/m^3		0.08 mg/m^3	x	1 mg/m^3	1 mg/m^3	1 mg/m^3
2-Nitrobiphenyl			(P)		(P)		(P)		x
4-Nitrobiphenyl	3	A1 (S)			(P)		x		
2-Nitropropane	2B	A2 10 ppm (36 mg/m^3)	10 ppm	20 ppm	8 ppm		25 ppm		10 ppm
N-Nitrosodimethylamine	2A	A2 (S)			(P)				x
Phenylhydrazine		A2 0.1 ppm (0.44 mg/m^3) (S)	5 ppm (S)				5 ppm (S)		5 ppm (S)
N-Phenyl-2-naphthylamine	3	A2							x
Polycyclic aromatic hydrocarbons (benzene-soluble fractions)			x				0.2 mg/m^3		0.2 mg/m^3
1,3-Propane sultone	2B	A2			(P)				x
β-Propiolactone	2B	A2 0.5 ppm (1.5 mg/m^3)	0.5 ppm						x
Propyleneimine	2B	A2 2 ppm (4.7 mg/m^3) (S)	2 ppm (S)	1.6 ppm (S)			2 ppm		2 ppm (S)
Tetrachloroethylene	2B	50 ppm (339 mg/m^3)	270 mg/m^3 (S)	525 mg/m^3 (S)	536 mg/m^3 (S)	670 mg/m^3	670 mg/m^3	1000 mg/m^3	670 mg/m^3 (S)
ortho-Toluidine	2B	A2 (S)	(S)						2 ppm
ortho-Toluidine	2B	A2 2 ppm (8.8 mg/m^3) (S)	2 ppm				5 ppm (S)		2 ppm
Trichloroethylene	3	50 ppm (269 mg/m^3)		420 mg/m^3	428 mg/m^3		535 mg/m^3		535 mg/m^3

Table 2 (contd)

Latin America

Agent	IARC (1993)	ACGIH (1991–92)	Argentina	Brazil	Chile	Cuba	Mexico	Peru	Venezuela
Vinyl bromide	2A	A2 5 ppm (22 mg/m3)							5 ppm
Vinyl chloride	1	A1 5 ppm (13 mg/m3)	5 ppm (398 mg/m3) (S)	156 ppm (C) (8 mg/m3)	4 ppm		10 ppm	1300 mg/m3	5 ppm
Vinylcyclohexene dioxide	3	A2 10 ppm (57 mg/m3) (S)	10 ppm (S)				10 ppm		10 ppm

Asia

Agent	IARC (1993)	ACGIH (1991–92)	China	Taiwan Province	Hong Kong	India	Indonesia	Republic of Korea	Philippines	Singapore	Thailand
Acetylaminofluorene	2A					(P)	(P)				
Acrylonitrile	1	A2 2 ppm (4.3 mg/m3) (S)	2 mg/m3 (S)	2 ppm (S)		2 ppm	20 ppm (S)	2 ppm	2 ppm		
4-Aminobiphenyl	1	A1 (S)		x	(P)		(P)				
Aniline	3	2 ppm (7.6 mg/m3) (S)	5 mg/m3 (S)	5 ppm (S)		2 ppm	5 ppm (S)				
Antimony trioxide production	2B	A2 0.5 mg/m3 (compound)					x				
Arsenic and compounds (As)	1	0.2 mg/m3 (soluble compound)	0.5 mg/m3		0.2 mg/m3	0.5 mg/m3			0.2 mg/m3		
Arsenic trioxide production (As)	1	A2						x			
Asbestos (all forms)	1	A1 0.2–2 f/cm3 [a]	2 f/cm3			0.2–2 f/cm3	1 f/cm3	x	2 f/cm3 >5µm	0.2–2 f/cm3	5 f/cm3
Asphalt fumes	3	5 mg/m3				5 mg/m3					
Auramine production	1				x						
Benzene (Benzol)	1	A2 10 ppm (32 mg/m3) [b]	40 mg/m3 (S)	25 ppm (S)		10 ppm	16 ppm	10 ppm		10 ppm	
Benzidine and its salts	1	A1 (S)	(P)	x	(P)		(P)				
Benzyl chloride	2B	1 ppm (5.2 mg/m3)							1 ppm		
Beryllium and compounds (Be)	1	A2 0.002 mg/m3	0.001 mg/m3	0.002 mg/m3		0.002 mg/m3	0.002 mg/m3	0.002 mg/m3			0.002 mg/m3
Bis(chloromethyl)ether	1	A1 0.001 ppm (0.0047 mg/m3)			0.001 ppm						
1,3-Butadiene	2A	A2 10 ppm (22 mg/m3)		1000 ppm			1000 ppm				
Cadmium and compounds (Cd)	1	0.05 mg/m3 [c]	0.1 mg/m3 (dust)		0.05 mg/m3 (dust)						
Cadmium oxide, production (Cd)	1	0.05 mg/m3	0.1 mg/m3 (fumes)								

Agent	IARC (1993)	ACGIH (1991–92)	Asia								
			China	Taiwan Province	Hong Kong	India	Indonesia	Republic of Korea	Philippines	Singapore	Thailand
Carbon tetrachloride	2B	A2 5 ppm (31 mg/m^3) (S)	25 mg/m^3 (S)	10 ppm (S)		10 ppm (S)	10 ppm	5 ppm	10 ppm		
Chloroform	2B	A2 10 ppm (49 mg/m^3)		50 ppm			50 ppm (C)	10 ppm			
Chloromethyl methyl ether	1	A2									
Chromate lead (Pb) (Cr)	1	A2 0.05 mg/m^3 (0.012 mg/m^3)									
Chromate zinc (Cr)	1	A1 0.01 mg/m^3									
Chromic acid (dichromic and salts (Cr)	1	0.05 mg/m^3				0.05 mg/m^3		x			
Chromite ore processing (Cr)		A1 0.05 mg/m^3							0.05 mg/m^3		
Chromium[VI] compounds (Cr)	1	A1 0.05 mg/m^3									
Chromium & compounds (Cr)		0.05–0.5 mg/m^3	0.05 mg/m^3	0.1 mg/m^3 (S)	0.05 mg/m^3	0.1 mg/m^3	0.05 mg/m^3				
Chrysene	3	A2									
Coal-tar pitch (volatile, soluble in benzene)	1	A1 0.2 mg/m^3		0.2 mg/m^3			0.2 mg/m^3		0.2 mg/m^3		
Dianisidine and salts	2B			x (ortho)	x			x			
para-Dichlorobenzene	2B	75 ppm (451 mg/m^3)^d		50 ppm			75 ppm				
3,3'-Dichlorobenzidine	2B	A2 (S)		x (ortho)	x		(P)	x			
Dimethylcarbamoyl chloride	2A	A2									
1,1-Dimethylhydrazine	2B	A2 0.5 ppm (1.2 mg/m^3)^e (S)	5 mg/m^3			1 mg/m^3	0.5 ppm (S)				
Dimethylsulfate	2A	A2 0.1 ppm (0.52 mg/m^3) (S)				5 mg/m^3	1 ppm (S)		1 ppm (S)		
Diphenylamine		10 mg/m^3					10 mg/m^3				
Ethylene dibromide	2A	A2 (S)					20 ppm (S/C)				
Ethyleneimine		0.5 ppm (0.88 mg/m^3) (S)		0.5 ppm (S)			0.5 ppm (S)	0.5 ppm			
Ethylene oxide	2A	A2 1 ppm (1.8 mg/m^3)		50 ppm			50 ppm				
Formaldehyde	2A	A2 1 ppm (1.2 mg/m^3)^f	3 mg/m^3	5 ppm (S)		1 ppm	5 ppm (C)			3 ppm	
Hexachloro-1,3-butadiene	3	A2 0.02 ppm (0.21 mg/m^3) (S)									
Hexamethylphosphoramide	2B	A2 (S)									
Hydrazine	2B	A2 0.1 ppm (0.13 mg/m^3)^g (S)	1.3 mg/m^3			1.3 mg/m^3	1 ppm (S)		1 ppm (S)		
Isopropanol manufacture (strong-acid process)	1	400 ppm (983 mg/m^3) (compound)		400 ppm							

Table 2 (contd)

Agent	IARC (1993)	ACGIH (1991–92)	Asia								
			China	Taiwan Province	Hong Kong	India	Indonesia	Republic of Korea	Philippines	Singapore	Thailand
Lead	2B	0.15 mg/m3	0.05 mg/m3 (fumes)	0.15 mg/m3		0.15 mg/m3	0.15 mg/m3				mg/m3
Magenta	2B									x	
Magenta production	1				x			x			
Methyl iodide	3	A2 2 ppm (12 mg/m3) (S)		5 ppm				2 ppm			
4,4'-Methylene bis(2-chloroaniline)	2A	A2 0.02 ppm (0.22 mg/m3)[h] (S)					x				
Methylene chloride	2B	A2 50 ppm (174 mg/m3)		500 ppm			250 ppm				
Methylhydrazine		A2 0.2 ppm (0.38 mg/m3)[i]					0.2 ppm (S/C)				
Naphthylamine				x	x			x			
2-Naphthylamine	1	A1		x	(P)		(P)				
Nickel carbonyl (Ni)	1	0.05 ppm (0.12 mg/m3)[j]	0.001 mg/m3	0.35 mg/m3		0.05 mg/m3	0.007 mg/m3		0.007		
Nickel sulfide (roast, fume, dust) (Ni)	1	A1 1 mg/m3[j]							10 mg/m3		mg/m3
Nickel compounds (Ni)	1	0.1–1 mg/m3[j]					1 mg/m3			1 mg/m3	
2-Nitrobiphenyl		A1 (S)		x			(P)				
4-Nitrobiphenyl	3	A1 (S)		x	(P)						
2-Nitropropane	2B	A2 10 ppm (36 mg/m3)					25 ppm				
N-Nitrosodimethylamine	2A	A2 (S)					(P)				
Phenylhydrazine	3	A2 0.1 ppm (0.44 mg/m3) (S)				22 mg/m3 (S)	(S)				
N-Phenyl-2-naphthylamine	3	A2									
Polychlorinated biphenyls	2A	A2						0.5 mg/m3			
1,3-Propane sultone	2B										
β-Propiolactone	2B	A2 0.5 ppm (1.5 mg/m3)		x			(P)	0.5 ppm			
Propyleneimine	2B	A2 2 ppm (4.7 mg/m3) (S)									
Tetrachloroethylene	2B	50 ppm (339 mg/m3)		100 ppm			100 ppm	50 ppm			
ortho-Tolidine	2B	A2 (S)		x							
ortho-Toluidine	2B	A2 2 ppm (8.8 mg/m3) (S)				2 ppm (S)	5 ppm (S)	2 ppm			
Trichloroethylene	3	50 ppm (269 mg/m3)	30 mg/m3	100 ppm	x	100 ppm	100 ppm	50 ppm			

Agent	IARC (1993)	ACGIH (1991–92)	Asia								
			China	Taiwan Province	Hong Kong	India	Indonesia	Republic of Korea	Philippines	Singapore	Thailand
Vinyl bromide	2A	A2 5 ppm (22 mg/m3)					250 ppm				
Vinyl chloride	1	A1 5 ppm (13 mg/m3)	30 mg/m3	10 ppm		5 ppm	1 ppm (C)	5 ppm	5 ppm	1 ppm	
Vinylcyclohexene dioxide	3	A2 10 ppm (57 mg/m3) (S)									

Agent	IARC (1993)	ACGIH (1991–92)	Middle East				
			Bahrain	Cyprus	Egypt	Iraq	Kuwait
Acetylaminofluorene					x		
Acrylonitrile	2A	A2 2 ppm (4.3 mg/m3)	2 ppm (S)		x	x	
4-Aminobiphenyl	1	A1 (S)				x	10 mg/m3
Aniline	3	2 ppm (7.6 mg/m3) (S)			x		
Arsenic and compounds (As)	1	0.2 mg/m3 (soluble compound)		0.01 mg/m3		x	0.5 mg/m3
Asbestos (all forms)	1	A1 0.2–2 f/cm3 [a]	0.2 f/cm3 (blue)	2 f/cm3	x	x	2 f/cm3
Asphalt fumes	3	5 mg/m3					5 mg/m3
Auramine production	1					x	
Benzene (Benzol)	1	A2 10 ppm (32 mg/m3)[b]	10 ppm	10 ppm	x	x	30 mg/m3
Benzidine and its salts	1	A1 (S)		x	x	x	
Benzyl chloride	2B	1 ppm (5.2 mg/m3)		0.002 mg/m3	x (salts)	x	
Beryllium and compounds (Be)	1	A2 0.002 mg/m3	0.002 mg/m3		x	x	
N,N'-Bis(2-chloroethyl)-2-naphthylamine (Chlornaphazine)	1						
Bis(chloromethyl)ether	1	A1 0.001 ppm (0.0047 mg/m3)	0.001 ppm			x	
Cadmium and compounds (Cd)	1	0.05 mg/m3 [c]		0.05 m/gm3		x	0.2 mg/m3
Cadmium oxide, production (Cd)	1	0.05 mg/m3 [c]	x				
Carbon tetrachloride	2B	A2 5 ppm (31 mg/m3) (S)	5 ppm		100 ppm	x	
Chlordane	2B	0.5 mg/m3 (S)	0.5 mg/m3				
Chlordimeform	3		x				
Chloroform	2B	A2 10 ppm (49 mg/m3)	10 ppm	10 ppm	x		
Chloromethyl methyl ether	1	A2	x				
Chromate lead (Pb) (Cr)	1	A2 0.05 mg/m3	0.05 mg/m3				
Chromate zinc (Cr)	1	A1 0.01 mg/m3	0.05 mg/m3				

Table 2 (contd)

Agent	IARC (1993)	ACGIH (1991–92)	Middle East				
			Bahrain	Cyprus	Egypt	Iraq	Kuwait
Chromite ore processing (Cr)		A1 0.05 mg/m³	0.05 mg/m³				
Chromium[VI] compounds (Cr)	1	A1 0.05 mg/m³					
Chromium and compounds (Cr)		0.05–0.5 mg/m³			0.1 mg/m³		0.05 mg/m³
Coal-tar pitch (volatile, soluble in benzene)	1	A1 0.2 mg/m³			x		0.2 mg/m³
DDT	2B	1 mg/m³	x	Banned			
para-Dichlorobenzene	2B	75 ppm (451 mg/m³)^d			75 ppm		
3,3′-Dichlorobenzidine	2B	A2 (S)	x				
Dieldrin	3	0.25 mg/m³ (S)	0.25 mg/m³ (S)				
para-Dimethylaminoazobenzene	2B	A2	x		x		
Dimethylcarbamoyl chloride	2A	A2	x				
1,1-Dimethylhydrazine	2B	A2 0.5 ppm (1.2 mg/m³)^e (S)	0.5 ppm			x	
Dimethylsulfate	2A	A2 0.1 ppm (0.52 mg/m³) (S)	0.1 ppm			x	
Diphenylamine		10 mg/m³			x		
Endrin	3	0.1 mg/m³ (S)	x				
Ethylene dibromide	2A	A2 (S)	x				
Ethylene oxide	2A	A2 1 ppm (1.8 mg/m³)	1 ppm	50 ppm	x	x	
Formaldehyde	2A	A2 1 ppm (1.2 mg/m³)^f	2 ppm		5 ppm	x	
Haematite mining (underground)	1					x	
Heptachlor	2B	0.5 mg/m³ (S)^k	x				
Hexachloro-1,3-butadiene	3	A2 0.02 ppm (0.21 mg/m³) (S)	0.02 ppm				
Hexamethyl phosphoric acid					x		
Hexamethylphosphoramide	2B	A2 (S)	x				
Hydrazine	2B	A2 0.1 ppm (0.13 mg/m³)^g (S)	0.1 ppm		x		
Isopropanol manufacture (strong acid process)	1					x	
Lead	2B	0.15 mg/m³		0.15 mg/m³	0.2 mg/m³		
Lindane	2B	0.5 mg/m³ (S)					
Methyl iodide	3	A2 2 ppm (12 mg/m³) (S)	2 ppm				
4,4′-Methylene bis(2-chloroaniline) (MOCA)	2A	A2 0.02 ppm (0.22 mg/m³)^h (S)	0.2 ppm				
Mirex	2B		x				
Mustard gas	1					x	

Agent	IARC (1993)	ACGIH (1991–92)	Middle East				
			Bahrain	Cyprus	Egypt	Iraq	Kuwait
Naphthylamine				x			
2-Naphthylamine	1	A1			x	x	
Nickel sulfide (roast, fume, dust)	1	A1 1 mg/m3 j	1.0 mg/m3				
Nickel compounds (Ni)	1	0.1–1 mg/m3 j		1.0 mg/m3		x	x
2-Nitrobiphenyl					x		
2-Nitropropane	2B	A2 10 ppm (36 mg/m3)	10 ppm				
Nitrosamines					x		
N-Nitrosodimethylamine	2A	A2 (S)	x				
Phenyl chloride/bromide					x		
Phenylhydrazine	3	A2 0.1 ppm (0.44 mg/m3) (S)	5 ppm		x		
N-Phenyl-2-naphthylamine	2A	A2	x			x	
Polychlorinated biphenyls			1 mg/m3				
Polycyclic aromatic hydrocarbons				x			
1,3-Propane sultone	2B	A2	x				
β-Propiolactone	2B	A2 0.5 ppm (1.5 mg/m3)	0.5 ppm				
Propyleneimine	2B	A2 2 ppm (4.7 mg/m3) (S)	2 ppm				
Tetrachloroethylene	2B	50 ppm (339 mg/m3)		100 ppm	5 ppm		
ortho-Tolidine	2B	A2 (S)	x				
ortho-Toluidine	2B	A2 2 ppm (8.8 mg/m3) (S)	2 ppm		x		
Trichloroethylene	3	50 ppm (269 mg/m3)			50 ppm		
Vinyl bromide	2A	A2 5 ppm (22 mg/m3)	5 ppm				
Vinyl chloride	1	A1 5 ppm (13 mg/m3)	5 ppm	x			
Vinylcyclohexene dioxide	3	A2 10 ppm (57 mg/m3) (S)	10 ppm				

(S), skin; blank, no information available; (P), prohibited; x, no time-weighted average given, substance only listed; (C), ceiling

IARC (1993), most recent evaluation in IARC Monographs

ACGIH (1991–92), evaluation of American Conference of Govermental Industrial Hygienists (1991). A1, confirmed human carcinogen, substance or substance associated with industrial processes recognized as having carcinogenic potential; A2, suspected human carcinogen, substance or substance associated with industrial process suspected of inducing cancer, on the basis of either limited epidemiological evidence or demonstration of carcinogenesis in one or more animal species by appropriate methods. Exposures to carcinogens must be kept to a minimum. Workers exposed to A1 carcinogens without a threshold limit value should be properly equipped to eliminate virtually all exposure to the carcinogen. For A1 carcinogens with a threshold limit value and for A2 carcinogens, exposures by all routes should be carefully controlled to levels as low as reasonably achievable below the threshold limit value.

a Intended change, 0.2 f/cm3 all forms; b Intended change, A1 0.1 ppm (0.3 mg/m3); c Intended changes, A2 0.01 mg/m3 (total dust); A2 0.002 mg/m3 (respirable fraction) ;
d Intended change, A2 10 ppm (60 mg/m3); e Intended change, A2 0.01 ppm (0.025 mg/m3); f Intended change, A2 0.3 ppm (0.37 mg/m3); g Intended change, A2 0.01 ppm (0.013 mg/m3) (S);
h Intended change, A1 (S); i Intended change, A2 0.01 ppm (0.019 mg/m3) (S); j Intended change, A1 0.05 mg/m3; k Intended change, A2 0.05 mg/m3

intermediates the carcinogenic agents and substances listed in an annex (Argentinian Government, 1990). Two separate resolutions establish rules for the use, handling and storage of polychlorinated biphenyls and for the use and handling of asbestos and asbestos wastes (Argentinian Government, 1991a,b). Decree 351/79 established maximum permissible concentrations for chemical pollutants, including chemical carcinogens. A regulation from 1990 created a registry of the enterprises that produce, import, use or obtain as intermediates the carcinogenic agents and substances listed in an annex to Decree 351/79 (Argentinian Government, 1991c). That list was modified by Regulation 444/91 of the Ministry of Work and Social Security in 1991 to include carcinogenic chemicals in two groups: A1 (confirmed carcinogens for humans) and A2 (suspected carcinogens for humans), as shown in Table 2 (Argentinian Government, 1991a).

Benin: Decree 93901 GTLS-HOF of 30 November 1955 establishes that safety and health measures be taken in industries in which workers could be intoxicated by benzene.

Brazil: The regulations are based on old ACGIH threshold limit values and have not been updated: The exposure limits are based on a 48-h work week, rather than on the 40-h work week assumed in US limits; several carcinogens, such as chromium compounds, are not regulated, and others are regulated less stringently (Frumkin & Câmara, 1991; Brazilian Government, 1991a). Substances with known threshold limit values (Cook, 1987) are also listed. The ILO Convention 162 (ILO, 1986) on asbestos, which was promulgated in 1991, fixes the permissible exposure level (PEL) for chrysotile fibres at 2 f/cm^3 and prohibits the employment of minors (under 18 years of age) when there is a possibility of exposure to asbestos (Brazilian Government, 1991b,c).

Chile: Decree 109, article 62 established three categories of carcinogens: proven, animal carcinogens (not proven in humans) and possible carcinogens. Maximum allowable concentrations (MAC) have been established (Chilean Government, 1983).

China: Document TJ3-79, promulgated in 1979, contains a MAC list of 88 substances (Cook, 1987). The MAC is defined as the concentration at or below which an acute or chronic occupational health effect should not occur in workers exposed for a long period. It is not a shift average concentration but a ceiling level that should not be exceeded in any representative sampling of airborne toxicants in the workplace. The Ministry of Public Health appointed a Standing Committee on Standard Setting in 1981. The standards are promulgated after approval by the Central Government. The usual approach for obtaining a scientific basis for setting standards is to use national field and epidemiological surveys integrated with laboratory experiments. Foreign standards that coincide with the special conditions in China may be adopted after analysis and the necessary verification (Gang, 1985). The use of benzidine was prohibited in 1976 because of its known carcinogenicity (Yu et al., 1990). Information on benzene included in Table 2 was taken from Yin et al. (1987), that on formaldehyde from Jiang and Zhang (1988) and that on asbestos dust in the workplace air from Huang (1990).

The Province of Taiwan follows the ACGIH threshold limit values. Eleven of the chemicals listed in Table 2 are recognized carcinogens, but the regulations make no special reference to their carcinogenicity (Cook, 1989).

Colombia: The list of carcinogens is identical to that of the ACGIH (Cook, 1987) and so is not included in Table 2. Colombia also has rules for the use and handling of pesticides issued under the Pesticides Law of 1979 (Colombian Government, 1990).

Cuba: Cuba generally follows the MAC values of the former USSR (El Batawi, 1986). In 1976, regulations were established on pesticides to protect approximately 250 000 agricultural workers (Alexander & Anderson, 1984). Limit values for chemicals in the air of working areas are established under Cuban norm number 10-01-63 of 1991.

Cyprus: In the Control of Factory Atmosphere and Dangerous Substances Regulations 1973 to 1986, issued under the Factories Law Cap. 134, a number of suspected carcinogens were assigned PELs, as listed in Table 2. There is a register for workers exposed to asbestos, free silica, benzene and pesticides. The PEL for asbestos was established as 2 f/cm^3 for all types through Amendment No. 1705 of 1981 (ILO, 1984).

Ecuador: The list of carcinogens is identical to that of the ACGIH (Cook, 1987) and is thus not presented in Table 2. Ecuador has regulations on the formulation, fabrication, importation, use and commercialization of pesticides for agricultural use (Ecuadorian Government, 1990)

Egypt: No special regulation exists for carcinogens (Cook, 1987).

Hong Kong: Regulations to control the presence and use of carcinogenic substances in industrial undertakings were established in 1986 and include a list of nine chemicals (Table 2). Use of four of them, 4-aminobiphenyl, benzidine and its salts, 2-naphthylamine and 4-nitrobiphenyl, and of any substance containing one or more of the chemicals (other than as a by-product of a chemical reaction and in a total concentration not exceeding 1%), is prohibited. Six other agents are considered to be controlled substances, and regulations with respect to industrial undertakings in which any person is employed are established. Health registers of people employed in connection with carcinogenic substances must be kept; employers must fill out a form for each employee and send it to the Commissioner for Labour, at the Labour Department, when the person stops work. The purpose of these regulations is to control the presence and use of carcinogenic substances in industrial undertakings and to safeguard the health of people employed in any manufacture, process or work involving carcinogenic substances (Cook, 1987; Government of Hong Kong, 1986).

India: The Directorate General Factory Advice Service and Labour Institutes stated that a schedule on prevention and control of hazards caused by carcinogenic substances has been formulated under Model Rule of the Factories Act, in which carcinogens were classified into three groups: prohibited, restricted and controlled substances. The Institute of Occupational Health in Ahmedabad states that no special regulation for carcinogens exists. Regulations covering dangerous or hazardous processes or operations and the handling, storage and transportation of dangerous or hazardous substances exist under the Factories Act 1948, Revised Factories Act 1987,

Mines Act 1932, Insecticides Act 1968 and Environment Protection Act 1986. PEL values, as in Cook (1987), are also included.

Indonesia: The eight carcinogens to which no exposure is permitted are listed in Table 2, and the PELs established for other carcinogenic substances are given (Cook, 1987). The standard concentration limit for amosite and chrysotile fibres is 1 f/cm^3 (ILO, 1984), and regulations on occupational safety and health have been established for the use of asbestos and pesticides (Indonesian Government, 1986a,b).

Iraq: Instruction No. 2 of the Ministry of Health concerning carcinogens is based on the list given in *IARC Monographs* Supplement 1 (IARC, 1979). Article 1 of the Instruction lists substances considered to be carcinogens (IARC Group 1), and Article 2 lists probable carcinogens (IARC Groups 2A and 2B); Article 3 gives instructions for regulating exposure of workers (Iraqi Government, 1987).

Mexico: Modification of Guideline No. 10 (Mexican Government, 1984) is a list of maximum permissible concentrations of chemicals in the workplace. It lists three classes of potential carcinogens with PELs similar to those of the ACGIH (Cook, 1987).

Morocco: No specific regulations have been made for the use or control of occupational carcinogens. A project is under consideration for recognition of the following occupational exposures as potentially carcinogenic: asbestos, nickel, arsenic, chromium and chromium compounds, wood dust, vinyl chloride and aromatic amines and their derivatives.

Nigeria: The PEL for asbestos was fixed at 2 f/cm^3 for all types of fibres by the 'Projet de recueil de directives pratiques' (ILO, 1984). No specific regulations have been made on carcinogens, but regulations exist on related issues, including the Hazardous Substances Decree (1989), the Poison and Drug Control Act (1976) and the Factories Decree (1987). Several international conventions are in use, although some are not ratified, including the ILO convention on asbestos, the WHO guideline on asbestos and the ACGIH guidelines on chemical hazards.

Peru: PELs were set for some carcinogens in workplaces in 1975 (Peruvian Ministry of Labour, 1991).

Singapore: The following agents are considered to be carcinogenic and are controlled at the workplace: asbestos, benzene, hardwood, vinyl chloride monomer, tar, pitch, creosote, arsenic and acrylonitrile (J. Jeyaratnam, personal communication). Some carcinogens are covered by the Poisons Act (1939, amended 1989) and the Poisons (Hazardous Substances) Rules (1986).

South Africa: The guideline for permissible exposure in asbestos mines was 45 f/cm^3 until 1975, when it was reduced to 12 f/cm^3. The current guidelines are five long fibres and 200 short fibres plus particles per cubic centimetre underground. The surface guideline was established as 5 f/cm^3 after December 1981. The time-weighted average exposure for vinyl chloride was established at 8 ppm. A draft of safety regulations, including limit values for 'high-risk substances' and distributed for comment in the *Government Gazette* on 3 June 1983, included asbestos, acrylonitrile, 4-aminobiphenyl, arsenic and its compounds, benzidine, cadmium and its compounds, ethylene dibromide, chromium and its compounds, crystalline silica, chloromethyl

methyl ether, lead and its compounds, mercury and its compounds, β-naphthylamine, 4-nitrobiphenyl and vinyl chloride (Cook, 1987).

Thailand: The Ministry of Public Health has followed the occupational health guidelines for chemical hazards of the US National Institute for Occupational Safety and Health and the US Occupational Safety and Health Administration and the ACGIH threshold limit values for establishing a list of carcinogens. The PEL for asbestos was regulated on 30 May 1977 at 5 f/cm^3 (ILO, 1984). Several laws concerning control of chemicals, such as the Toxic Substances Control Act BE. 2510 (1977), deal with the manufacture, handling, storage, transport, advertising, labelling, sale and export of toxic substances; the Hazardous Substances Act BE 2535 (1992) covers further groups of hazardous substances.

Turkey: No special regulations have been made on carcinogens, but MAC values have been established for various chemicals in the Occupational Health and Safety Regulations. Exposure to asbestos dust in mines and quarries during the construction of tunnels is controlled (Turkish Government, 1990).

United Republic of Tanzania: The Occupational Health Services Act 1986 stipulates that any worker exposed to silica dust must undergo an annual medical examination, including a full chest X-ray (Riwa, 1990). This requirement appears, however, to apply only to currently exposed workers.

Venezuela: The country follows the ACGIH threshold limit values (Cook, 1987). Standards were established in 1985 for several carcinogens (Venezuelan Government, 1985).

Zambia: The PEL for asbestos was regulated on 1 May 1984 at 0.2 f/cm^3 for amosite and crocidolite, 0.5 f/cm^3 for chrysotile and 1 f/cm^3 for other varieties (ILO, 1984).

Zimbabwe: There is no comprehensive legislation on asbestos; instead, it is covered by general regulations on control of dust emissions and on pneumoconiosis. Since 1985, the maximum permissible quantity of chrysotile asbestos dust in the workplace air was set at 2 f/cm^3 for 4 h (Baloyi, 1989). No specific regulations are set on carcinogens, but chemical safety in general is regulated, and there is a pesticides register.

Occupational diseases recognized as being caused by chemicals

Table 3 lists the cancers and related diseases that are recognized as being of occupational origin in selected developing countries. The information is based primarily on responses to the IARC survey (see Appendix). Once again, the Table is not comprehensive but provides relevant examples of current practices.

Many countries legislate on carcinogens or on diseases produced by carcinogens, although very little is known about the incidence or prevalence of the diseases. As shown in Table 3, silicosis and asbestosis are the most generally recognized diseases, but they are rarely compensated. For example, of 1239 cases of silicosis in India identified over 40 years, only 80 were compensated. Limited data are available on occupational cancer.

Brazil: A list has been established of causes of occupational diseases, which includes arsenic, asbestos, benzene, its homologues and nitro and amino derivatives, beryllium, cadmium, chromium and its compounds, ionizing radiation, lead, silica

Table 3. Cancers and diseases recognized as being of occupational origin in selected countries and regions

Country or region	Disease								Reference
	Pneumo-coniosis	Silicosis	Asbestosis	Mesothe-lioma	Lung cancer	Bladder cancer	Leukaemia/lymphoma	Other cancers	
Angola	No	No	No	No	No	No	No	No	IARC survey
Bahrain	No	No	No	No	No	No	No	No	IARC survey
Benin	No	No	No	No	No	No	No	No	IARC survey
Botswana	No	No	No	Yes	No	No	No	No	IARC survey
Brazil	Yes	–	Yes	No	No	No	No	No	IARC survey
Cameroon	Yes	Yes	Yes	No	Yes	Yes	Yes	Skin (primary epithelioma)[a]	IARC survey
Chile	Yes	Yes	Yes	Yes	Yes	Yes	Yes	Skin	IARC survey
Colombia	–	Yes	Yes	Yes	Yes	Yes	–	Several[b]	Colombian Government (1987)
Costa Rica	No	No	No	No	No	No	No	No	IARC survey
Cuba	Yes	Yes	Yes	No	No	No	No	No	IARC survey
Cyprus	Yes	–	Yes	Yes	No	No	No	No	IARC survey
Egypt	Yes	Yes	Yes	Yes	Yes	No	No	Cancer[c]	IARC survey
Ethiopia	No	No	No	No	No	No	No	No	IARC survey
Guatemala	No	No	No	No	No	No	No	No	IARC survey
Hong Kong	Yes	Yes	Yes	–	–	Yes	–	Nasal cavity/sinus	Ng (1986)
India	Yes	Yes	Yes	Yes	Yes	Yes	Yes	Skin	IARC survey
Indonesia	Yes	–	–	–	–	–	–	–	Indonesian Government (1981)
Kuwait	–	Yes	Yes	Yes	Yes	Yes	Yes	Skin (basal-cell carcinoma)[d]	IARC survey
Mongolia	Yes	Yes	No	No	Yes	No	No	No	IARC survey

Table 3 (contd)

Country or region	Disease								Reference
	Pneumo-coniosis	Silicosis	Asbestosis	Mesothe-lioma	Lung cancer	Bladder cancer	Leukaemia/ lymphoma	Other cancers	
Morocco	Yes	Yes	Yes	No	No	No	Yes[e]	Skin (primary epithelioma)[a]	IARC survey
Nigeria	Yes	Yes	Yes	Yes	Yes	Yes	Yes	No	IARC survey
Peru	–	Yes	Yes	No	Yes	No	Yes	No	IARC survey
Philippines	–	Yes	Yes	No	No	No	No	74 unspecified[f]	IARC survey
Singapore	Yes	Yes	Yes	Yes				Liver	Chia *et al.* (1991)
South Africa	–	–	Yes	Yes	Yes	–	–	–	Myers (1981); Solomons (1984)
Thailand	Yes	Yes	Yes	Yes	Yes	Yes	Yes	No	IARC survey
Turkey	–	Yes	Yes	Yes	Yes	Yes	Yes	No	IARC survey
United Republic of Tanzania	Yes	Yes	Yes	Yes	Yes	Yes	Yes	Skin	IARC survey
Zimbabwe	Yes	–	Yes	–	–	–	–	–	Baloyi (1989); Cullen & Baloyi (1991)

–, no data available

[a] When produced by coal-tar

[b] Cancers of the scrotum and nasal sinus, hepatic angiosarcoma, carcinomas and precancerous lesions of the skin related to specific exposures

[c] Cancer as a 'complication of an occupational disease as asbestosis, chronic ulceration, etc'

[d] One basal-cell carcinoma of the skin was recognized and compensated in 1978.

[e] Leukemias when an exposure was to benzene and derivatives, skin when exposure was to oil or petroleum derivatives

[f] Cancers recognized by Employees Compensation Commission, January–November 1991

dust, tar, asphalt, paraffin and related materials. There are, however, no data on cancer as an occupational disease (Frumkin & Câmara, 1991).

Cameroon: The following occupational diseases are recognized; the time period for which the employer or the insurance body remains responsible for them is given in parentheses: leukosis (10 years), leukaemic conditions (3 years), leukopenia with neutropenia (1 year), slight, progressive anaemia of the hypoplastic or aplastic type (1 year) produced by benzene and its homologues such as xylene and toluene (No. 6677 5/10/56); leukosis (1 year), leukaemic conditions (10 years), leukopenia with neutropenia (1 year), slight, progressive anaemia of the hypoplastic or aplastic type (1 year), severe, progressive anaemia of the hypoplastic type (3 years), bone sarcoma (15 years) and lung cancer (10 years) produced by X-rays or radioactive substances (No. 6679, 5/10 56); bladder cancers produced by aromatic amines, mainly naphthylamine and benzidine (15 years) (No. 005, 9/03/62); primary epitheliomas of the skin produced by coal-tar and silicosis (No. 005, 9/03/62). Two cases of lymphoma/leukaemia (not specified) have been compensated.

Chile: Decree No. 71, Law 16744 refers to pneumoconiosis and establishes that a worker who presents radiological evidence of pneumoconiosis has the right to be compensated for 25% of his or her earnings (Prenafeta, 1984).

Colombia: Silicosis, asbestosis and diseases caused by cadmium and arsenic and its compounds are recognized as occupational diseases. A chapter in the Decree that refers to occupational cancer includes: cancer of the lung produced by occupational exposure to arsenic, radon, asbestos, chromium, nickel, bis(chloromethyl) ether or chloromethyl methyl ether; mesothelioma (pleural and peritoneal) produced by asbestos; cancer of the scrotum in printers produced by polycyclic aromatic hydrocarbons; cancer of the nasal sinus produced by exposure to nickel and isopropanol; hepatic angiosarcoma produced during production of polyvinyl chloride; bladder cancer in workers exposed to benzidine and 2-naphthylamine in dye production; carcinomas and precancerous lesions of the skin produced in workers handling tar, pitch, mineral oils and bitumen and its products and residues (Colombian Government, 1987)

Cuba: Asbestosis and silicosis are recognized as occupational diseases. Cancer will be recognized in the future by the Project of Ministry Resolution No. 34.

Cyprus: Five cases of asbestosis (period not stated) and 15 mesotheliomas (1986–92) had been recognized but not compensated.

Egypt: Asbestosis and silicosis are recognized as occupational diseases; cancer is recognized as a 'complication of an occupational disease'.

Hong Kong: Voluntary notification of silicosis began in 1956; compensation started in 1981, when a statutory scheme for compensation came into effect (Ng *et al.*, 1990). Pneumoconiosis is compensated under the Pneumoconiosis (Compensation) (Amendment) Ordinance 1980 (Government of Hong Kong, 1980). Asbestosis was included in the list of notifiable compensatable diseases in 1980 (Lam *et al.*, 1983), and 11 cases of asbestosis were recognized and compensated during the period 1986–90 (Government of Hong Kong, 1991). Of the 103 cases of pneumoconiosis compensated by the Pneumoconiosis Compensation Fund Board between 1986 and 1990, 97 had a history of employment in construction or quarrying, one in shipbuilding, two in jade polishing and one in mining. The asbestosis cases compensated during 1986–90 included seven workers with a history of employment in shipbuilding and repair, one mechanical technician, one vehicle mechanic, one seaman involved in maintenance mechanics and one foundry worker (Government of Hong Kong, 1991). An amendment to the Employees' Compensation Ordinance added tumours of the urinary tract due to occupational exposure to carcinogenic aromatic amines to the list of occupational diseases (Government of Hong Kong, 1987).

India: Asbestosis and silicosis are recognized in India as occupational diseases and are compensated. Forty-four cases of asbestosis were recognized in 2351 workers surveyed in the period 1985–90, and 26 were compensated; 1239 cases of silicosis were recognized in 1949–89 among 12 996 workers examined, and 80 were compensated. According to the Ministry of Labour, Directorate General Factory Advice Service and Labour Institutes, lung cancer, mesothelioma, bladder cancer, leukaemias and lymphomas and skin cancers are also recognized and compensatable, but the numbers of cases were not given.

Indonesia: Obligatory reporting has been established of occupational diseases, including those caused by beryllium, cadmium, chromium, arsenic, lead, carbon disulfide and benzene; pneumoconiosis caused by mineral dust; diseases of the lung and respiratory tract caused by solid metal dusts; and epitheliomas of the skin caused by tar, pitch, bitumen, mineral oil, anthracene or its compounds, products or residues (Indonesian Government, 1981).

Kuwait: Asbestosis, silicosis, cancer of the lung, mesothelioma, bladder cancer, leukaemia, lymphoma and other cancers are recognized as occupational diseases if an arbitration board determines a causal relationship. The current scheme compensates asbestosis only on the basis of decreased respiratory capacity. The one case compensated was in a man who had worked for nine years in mixing, with exposure to asbestos fibre, and in manufacturing, with exposure to asbestos–cement in a pipe factory (Mohamed, 1990).

Mexico: A technical standard for epidemiological monitoring of occupational health must be observed in all workplaces and health centres; pneumoconiosis (silicosis and asbestosis) and cancer are covered (Mexican Government, 1987).

Mongolia: Pneumoconiosis, silicosis and lung cancer are recognized as occupational diseases. In 1981–91, 2092 cases of pneumoconiosis, 841 cases of silicosis and 252 cases of lung cancer were recognized.

Morocco: The list of recognized occupational diseases includes pneumoconiosis, specifying silicosis and asbestosis, and complications of the latter. Leukaemias related to exposure to benzene and its nitro and amino derivatives and primary skin epitheliomas are also considered to be occupational diseases. In 1988, 299 cases of pneumoconiosis and eight cases of asbestosis were notified to the Ministry of Employment. The Medical Occupational Inspection Board registered 80 cases of asbestosis during 1970–92. A review of the files found 58 cases of asbestosis, all in the same asbestos–cement industry; they were associated with two cases of mesothelioma, three of bronchial cancer and one of oesophageal cancer (Alibou, 1990).

Mozambique: Medical conditions that result from occupational exposure to ambient asbestos or to dust from products containing asbestos are considered to be occupational illnesses (Mozambican Government, 1987).

Philippines: Asbestosis, silicosis and cancer are recognized as occupational diseases. Ninety-two cases of silicosis were observed among a population of workers involved in mining, ceramics and glass manufacture and in a cement establishment that was surveyed to determine the prevalence of pneumoconiosis (Chipongian et al., 1989). Seventy-four cases of cancer (without specifying site) were recognized by the Employees' Compensation Commission in January–November 1991.

Republic of Korea: Workers currently exposed to asbestos are required to undergo medical examinations. Screening, including a physical examination, chest X-ray and some laboratory tests if indicated, is inadequate owing to lack of qualified personnel and equipment. Access to workplaces, while guaranteed by law, is often difficult in practice, and employers often do not comply with regulations and inspectors' orders (Johannig et al., 1991).

Singapore: Asbestosis, arsenical poisoning, chronic benzene poisoning, epitheliomatous ulceration, liver angiosarcoma, toxic hepatitis and mesothelioma are notifiable diseases under the Factories Act. A register of all confirmed cases is maintained by the Department of Industrial Health, Ministry of Labour (Ho et al., 1987).

South Africa: Asbestosis, mesothelioma and lung cancer are compensatable diseases. Analysis of data on certificates of compensated diseases during 1977–78, by race, showed that 92% of the asbestos mine labour force was African; 57% of the asbestos-related disease certificates were for blacks and 43% for whites (Myers, 1981). Mesothelioma is a notifiable medical condition under the Health Act (Davies, 1986). It was classified as a compensatable occupational disease in the non-mining sector in 1979, although it has been compensated in the mining industry since 1962. The total number of cases during 1977–83 was reported to be 509 (Solomons, 1984); over the three-year period 1980–82, 78 cases of mesothelioma were diagnosed and compensated by the Medical Bureau for Occupational Diseases.

Thailand: Recognized occupational diseases include pneumoconiosis, asbestosis, byssinosis and diseases produced by exposure to arsenic, lead, benzene, carbon disulfide, chromium and its compounds, beryllium and carbon tetrachloride (Thai Government, 1972). Forty cases of asbestosis were recognized in the period 1977–89 but were not compensated.

Turkey: One case of asbestosis was recognized and compensated in 1990.

Zimbabwe: Zimbabwe has had a Pneumoconiosis Bureau since 1949. In 1984, a law was passed requiring universal surveillance of miners and others in 'dusty trades'—primarily people directly associated with mines. Cases of mesothelioma and lung cancer were found among Zimbabwean miners and millers, but neither disease has been listed formally as a compensatable disorder (Cullen & Baloyi, 1991). Since 1980, 51 individuals with asbestos exposure have been compensated for asbestos-related disease (Baloyi, 1989).

Conclusions

The existence of national lists of occupational carcinogens, usually derived from international lists, does not guarantee that occupational carcinogens are adequately controlled. Many countries have legislation on occupational cancer, and have even ratified the ILO Convention 139, but are in fact not aware of the problem of occupational cancer. Thus, although the existence of legislation is an important step in the prevention of occupational cancers it is not usually translated into better recognition and prevention.

References

Alexander, R. & Anderson, P.K. (1984) Pesticide use, alternatives and workers' health in Cuba. *Int. J. Health Serv.*, **14**, 31–41

Alibou, N. (1990) *L'Asbestose Respiratoire à propos de 58 Cas Coligés à l'Hôpital 20 Août de Casablanca de 1970 à 1988* [Respiratory asbestosis in 58 cases collected at the 20 August Hospital in Casablanca from 1970 to 1988], No. 1, Thesis, Casablanca

American Conference of Governmental Industrial Hygienists (1991) *TLVs Threshold Limit Values for Chemical Substances and Physical Agents and Biological Exposure Indices for 1991–1992*, Cincinnati, OH

Argentinian Government (1990) Regulation No. 33/90. *Bol. Of.*, **1 April**

Argentinian Government (1991a) *Salud Occupacional IX, No. 44:8–22 y No. 45:14–22. Concentraciones Maximas Permisibles para Contaminantes* [Occupational health IX, No. 44:8–22 and No. 45:14–22. Maximal permissible concentrations of contaminants] (Resolution 444/91), Buenos Aires

Argentinian Government (1991b) Resolution No. 369/91. *Bol. Of.*, **2 May**

Argentinian Government (1991c) Resolution No. 577/91. *Bol. Of.*, **16 July**

Baloyi, R. (1989) *Exposure to Asbestos among Chrysotile Miners, Millers and Mine Residents and Asbestosis in Zimbabwe*, Helsinki, Institute of Occupational Health

Brazilian Government (1991a) Decree No. 4. *Diario Of.*, **153**, 16110–16112

Brazilian Government (1991b) Decree No. 126. *Diario Of.*, **98**, 9778–9780

Brazilian Government (1991c) Regulation No. 01 of 28 May 1991, modifying Annex No. 1 of Standard No. 15 concerning 'Permissible levels for mineral dust' — asbestos (Brazil.). *Diario Of.*, **129**, 10191–10193 (in Portuguese)

Chia, S.-E., Chia, K.-S., Phoon, W.-H. & Lee, H.-P. (1991) Silicosis and lung cancer among Chinese granite workers. *Scand. J. Work Environ. Health*, **17**, 170–174

Chilean Government (1983) *Presidential Decree, 9 February*, Santiago

Chipongian, N.S., Castro, F.T., Somera-Cucueco, Ma,T., Yu-Sison, S., Reyes, R.P., Villanueva, M.B.G. & Ortega, V.S.D. (1989) A prevalence study of pneumoconiosis in four industrial establishments. Department of Labour and Employment, Quezon, Philippines (unpublished manuscript)

Colombian Government (1987) Decree No. 778 of 30 April 1987 amending the list of occupational diseases contained in Section 201 of the Basic Labour Code. *Diario Of.*, **37868**, 11–12 (in Spanish)

Colombian Government (1990) Decree No. 775. *Diario Of.*, **39300**, 12–23 (in Spanish)

Commission for the Investigation of Health Hazards of Chemical Compounds in the Work Area (1991) *Maximum Concentrations at the Workplace and Biological Tolerance Values for Working Materials* (Report No. 27), Weinheim, Deutsche Forschungsgemeinschaft, VHC

Cook, W.A. (1987) *Occupational Exposure Limits — Worldwide*, Akron, OH, American Industrial Hygiene Association

Cook, W.A. (1989) Occupational exposure limits for carcinogens — variant approaches by different countries. *Am. Ind. Hyg. Assoc. J.*, **50**, A-680–A-684

Cullen, M.R. & Baloyi, R.S. (1991) Chrysotile asbestos and health in Zimbabwe: I. Analysis of miners and millers compensated for asbestos-related diseases since independence (1980). *Am. J. Ind. Med.*, **19**, 161–169

Davies, J.C.A. (1986) Uncommon occupational diseases should be notified. *S.A. Med. J.*, **69**, 79–80

Ecuadorian Government (1990) Law No. 73. *Regist. Of.*, **442**, 2–6 (in Spanish)

El Batawi, M.A. (1986) The third Theodore F. Hatch symposium lecture. *Ann. Am. Conf. Gov. Ind. Hyg.*, **14**, 3–15

Frumkin, H. & Cämara, V.deM. (1991) Occupational health and safety in Brazil. *Am. J. Public Health*, **81**, 1619–1624

Gang, B.-Q. (1985) Development of occupational hygiene standards in the People's Republic of China. *Scand. J. Work Environ. Health*, **11** (Suppl. 4), 10–12

Government of Hong Kong (1980) Pneumoconiosis (Compensation) Ordinance No. 51 of 1980. *Hong Kong Gov. Gaz.*, A255–77

Government of Hong Kong (1986) *Laws of Hong Kong*, Chapter 360, *Pneumoconiosis (Compensation) Ordinance*, rev. ed. (Ordinance No. 51 of 1980), Hong Kong, Government Printer

Government of Hong Kong (1987) *The Employees' Compensation Ordinance* (Amendment of Second Schedule) *Order 1987. L.N. 52 of 1987.* Dated 17 February 1987. *Hong Kong Gov. Gaz.*, **129** (Legal Suppl. No. 2 to No. 9), B140–B141

Government of Hong Kong (1991) *Pneumoconiosis Compensation Fund Board Publication*

Ho, S.-F., Lee, H.-P. & Phoon, W.H. (1987) Malignant mesothelioma in Singapore. *Br. J. Ind. Med.*, **44**, 788–789

Huang, J.Q. (1990) A study on the dose–response relationship between asbestos exposure level and asbestosis among workers in a Chinese chrysotile product factory. *Biomed. Environ. Sci.*, **3**, 90–98

IARC (1979) *IARC Monographs on the Evaluation of the Carcinogenic Risk of Chemicals to Humans*, Suppl. 1, *Chemicals and Industrial Processes Associated with Cancer in Humans* (IARC Monographs, Volumes 1 to 20), Lyon

IARC (1993) *IARC Monographs on the Evaluation of Carcinogenic Risks to Humans, List of IARC Evaluations*, Lyon

ILO (1974) *Occupational Cancer Convention 139*, Geneva

ILO (1983) *Encyclopaedia on Occupational Safety and Health*, 3rd ed., Geneva

ILO (1984) *Securité dans l'Utilisation de l'Amiante* [Safety in the Use of Asbestos], Geneva

ILO (1986) *Asbestos Convention 162*, Geneva

ILO (1988) *Occupational Cancer: Prevention and Control*, Geneva

Indonesian Government (1981) *Decree on the Obligatory Reporting of Occupational Diseases* (No. PER-01/MEN/1981), Jakarta, Minister of Manpower and Transmigration

Indonesian Government (1986a) Regulation No. PER-03/MEN/1985. *Labour Legis. Indonesia*, **3**, 11–15

Indonesian Government (1986b) Regulation No. PER-03/MEN/1986 on safety and health conditions in work sites managing pesticides. *Labour Legis. Indonesia*, **3** (Suppl.), 60–63

Iraqi Government (1987) *Rapport Presenté par le Governement Iraquien au Sujet de la Convention No. 139 de 1974 pour la Periode se Terminant le 30 Juin 1991* [Report presented by the Iraqi Government concerning Convention No. 139 for the period ending 30 June 1991], Baghdad

Jiang, X.-Z. & Zhang, R.-W. (1988) The toxicity and potential risk of occupational exposure to formaldehyde. In: Xue, S.-Z. & Liang, Y.-X., eds, *Occupational Health in Industrialization and Modernization* (Bulletin of WHO Collaborating Center for Occupational Health, Shanghai, Vol. 2), Shanghai, Shanghai Medical University Press, pp. 70–74

Johannig, E., Selikoff, I.J. & Goldberg, M. (1991) *Asbestos Health Hazard Evaluation in South Korea. Asbestos Textile Manufacturing*, New York, Mount Sinai Medical Center

Lam, W.K., Kung, T.M., Ma, P.L., So, S.Y. & Mok, C.K. (1983) First report of asbestos-related disease in Hong Kong. *Trop. Geogr. Med.*, **35**, 225–229

Mexican Government (1984) Modifications to Instructivo No. 10. *Diario Of.*, **28 May** (in Spanish)

Mexican Government (1987) Technical Standard No. 79. *Diario Of.*, **7**, 11–17 (in Spanish)

Mohamed, I.Y. (1990) Asbestos–cement pneumoconiosis: first surgically confirmed case in Kuwait. *Am. J. Ind. Med.*, **17**, 241–245

Mozambican Government (1987) Act No. 8 of 14 December 1985. *Bol. Repub.*, **50** (Suppl. 5), 196 (in Portuguese)

Myers, J. (1981) The social context of occupational disease: asbestos and South Africa. *Int. J. Health Serv.*, **11**, 227–245

Ng, T.P. (1986) A case–referent study of cancer of the nasal cavity and sinuses in Hong Kong. *Int. J. Epidemiol.*, **15**, 171–175

Ng, T.P., Chan, S.L. & Lee, J. (1990) Mortality of a cohort of men in a silicosis register: further evidence of an association with lung cancer. *Am. J. Ind. Med.*, **17**, 163–171

Peruvian Ministry of Labour (1991) *Decree Supreme No. 00258-75-SA, 22 September 1975*, Lima (in Spanish)

Prenafeta, J. (1984) Pneumoconiosis in Chile. *Rev. Méd. Chile*, **112**, 511–515 (in Spanish)

Riwa, P.D. (1990) Silicosis: a problem of our times too. *Afr. Newslett. Occup. Health Saf.*, **31 August**, 8–9

Rothwell, K. (1992) *The Interaction of Smoking and Workplace Hazards. Risks to Health* (WHO/OCH/TOH/92.1), Geneva, WHO

Solomons, K. (1984) Malignant mesothelioma—clinical and epidemiological features. A report of 80 cases. *S. Afr. Med. J.*, **66**, 407–412

Thai Government (1972) *Government Gazette*, **89** (Part 61), BE 2515 (in Thai)

Turkish Government (1990) Regulation of the Ministry of Labour and Safety. *Resmi Gaz.*, **20635**, 12–21 (in Turkish)

Venezuelan Government (1985) Resolution No. 187. *Gac. Of.*, **33185**, 352785–352786 (in Spanish)

WHO (1980) *Recommended Health-based Limits in Occupational Exposure to Heavy Metals. Report of a WHO Study Group* (Technical Report Series 647), Geneva

WHO (1981) *Recommended Health-based Limits in Occupational Exposure to Selected Organic Solvents. Report of a WHO Study Group* (Technical Report Series 664), Geneva

WHO (1982) *Recommended Health-based Limits in Occupational Exposure to Pesticides. Report of a WHO Study Group* (Technical Report Series 677), Geneva

WHO (1986) *Early Detection of Occupational Diseases*, Geneva

WHO (1987) *Eighth General Programme of Work Covering the Period 1990–1995*, Geneva

WHO/EURO (1990) *Occupational Health Services. Report of a WHO Consultation, Helsinki, 22–24 May 1989* (EUR/ICP/OCH/134), Copenhagen

WHO/EURO (1991) *Lifestyle and Health Risks at the Workplace* (European Occupational Health Series No. 3), Copenhagen

Yin, S.-N., Li, Q., Liu, Y., Tian, F., Du, C. & Jin, C. (1987) Occupational exposure to benzene in China. *Br. J. Ind. Med.*, **44**, 192–195

Yu, M.C., Garabrant, D.H., Huang, T.-B. & Henderson, B.E. (1990) Occupational and other non-dietary risk factors for nasopharyngeal carcinoma in Guangzhou, China. *Int. J. Cancer*, **45**, 1033–1039

Chapter 10. Strategies for the Prevention of Occupational Cancer in Developing Countries

N. Pearce and E. Matos

Introduction

It is often argued (e.g. Doll & Peto, 1981) that occupational exposures do not account for a high proportion of cancer cases. Occupational carcinogens are nevertheless very important in public health terms, because occupational exposures can be prevented or minimized relatively more easily than general life-style factors such as tobacco, diet, sexual practices and exposure to sunlight. Furthermore, prevention of occupational exposures often also prevents environmental exposures. Although there are few well-documented examples, even in industrialized countries, of a reduction in cancer risk following the elimination of a carcinogenic occupational exposure (Swerdlow, 1990), such reductions may be assumed to have occurred frequently as permissible exposure levels to recognized carcinogens have been reduced. Occupational cancer is therefore not an unavoidable burden but should be regarded as an indicator of the distorted, self-limiting development of some branches of industry (Simonato, 1986).

The greatest advances in prevention of cancer in industrialized countries have been the result of political and economic changes rather than of prevention at the level of individual exposures to specific agents. The same principles are likely to apply in developing countries. For example, the health effects of tobacco smoking have been known for several decades; attempts at prevention at the individual level have had some success in higher-income groups but have had little success in other sections of the community (Pearce *et al.*, 1985). More effective legislative measures (such as advertising bans, price increases and limits on smoking in public places) have been adopted in recent years, although these measures have still tended to focus on tobacco consumption rather than on the problem of tobacco production. Thus, the industry has shifted its promotional activities to developing countries (Tominaga, 1986), so that more people are exposed to tobacco smoke than ever before. In most instances, developing countries lack the political and economic strength needed to impose the kinds of restrictions that are increasingly being adopted in western countries. The inequalities in health between industrialized and developing countries are therefore increasing.

Some parallels can be drawn with production processes that are associated with cancer. These are also being increasingly regulated in industrialized countries and are consequently being transferred to developing countries. Once again, although local initiatives (e.g. in individual factories and industries) may have some preventive effect, the greatest impact is likely to come from the establishment and enforcement of national and international regulatory controls. Again, however, most developing countries lack the political and economic strength to impose such controls, particularly since worker organizations are generally weak (Michaels *et al.*, 1985; Elling, 1988). The situation is made much more difficult by the current debt crisis of many developing countries (see Chapter 2). Furthermore, many developing countries are suffering from the effects of extreme structural adjustment programmes, mandated by the World Bank, which are increasing unemployment and reducing access to health care (Logie & Woodroffe, 1993).

Some progress can be made in the prevention of occupational cancer, even in the current international situation. In the following sections, we review general strategies for the prevention of occupational cancer in developing countries, discuss international regulatory efforts and draw some general conclusions.

General strategies for the prevention of occupational cancer

Swerdlow (1990) outlined a series of options for the prevention of exposure to occupational causes of cancer.

Non-introduction of carcinogens into the workplace

The most successful form of prevention is to avoid use of recognized human carcinogens in the workplace. This has rarely, if ever, been an option in industrialized countries: virtually all occupational carcinogens have been identified as such by epidemiological studies of populations that were already occupationally exposed. Nevertheless, there are some examples of carcinogens that were used in certain industrialized countries but not in others. For example, 4-aminobiphenyl (xenylamine), a potent bladder carcinogen, was used in the USA but was never manufactured commercially or widely used in the United Kingdom because of concern that it would prove to be carcinogenic (Swerdlow, 1990).

In theory, developing countries could learn from the experience of industrialized countries and prevent the introduction of chemicals and production processes that have been found to be hazardous. Such 'primordial prevention' rarely occurs, however, because most developing countries lack the political and economic strength to impose controls. Instead, as discussed in Chapter 2, hazardous industries tend to be transferred deliberately to developing countries in order to avoid regulatory control. International efforts to prevent and control such transfer are now being developed (see below).

Removal of carcinogens

The next best option after non-introduction of established carcinogens is removal of such agents once their carcinogenicity has been established or suspected. Once again, relatively few examples exist; they include the closure of plants making the bladder carcinogens α-naphthylamine and benzidine in the United Kingdom (Anon., 1965); termination of British gas manufacture involving coal carbonization; closure of Japanese and British mustard gas factories after the end of the Second World War (Swerdlow, 1990); and gradual elimination of the use of benzene in the shoe industry in Istanbul (Aksoy, 1985). Even fewer examples exist in developing countries of complete removal of occupational carcinogens. One such example was reported by Yin *et al.* (1987): A 1.9% incidence of aplastic anaemia was found in a Chinese shoemaking factory, and four cases of aplastic anaemia were detected among 211 workers over an eight-month period; exposure to benzene was estimated to be very high (daily mean concentration, about 1035.6 mg/m^3). As a result, production was stopped. A new solvent containing no benzene was introduced, and no further case developed.

Reduction in exposure levels

In many other instances, however, complete removal of a carcinogen (without closing down the industry) is either not possible (because alternative, noncarcinogenic agents are not available) or is judged politically or economically unacceptable (because the alternative agents are more expensive). Exposure levels must therefore be reduced by changing production processes and industrial hygiene practices, as has occurred in many industrialized countries in recent decades. Exposures to recognized carcinogens, such as asbestos, nickel, arsenic, benzene, pesticides and ionizing radiation, have progressively been reduced.

A number of similar examples have been seen in developing countries. For example, regulations on safety standards and surveillance of miners to ensure healthy working conditions were established in Zimbabwe in 1984 (see Chapter 9). Mechanical systems involving a negative pressure system with large main fans located on the surface have been installed in mines to ensure adequate ventilation. New mills have been built to ensure, as far as possible, that the milling and blending of asbestos is nearly totally enclosed. Dusty plants still exist, however (Ushewokunze, 1982).

Reduction in hazardous activities

A related approach is to reduce or eliminate the activities that involve the heaviest exposures. For example, 65 years after Pott reported the existence of scrotal cancer in chimney sweeps, in 1775, an act was passed in England and Wales to prohibit chimney sweeps from being sent up chimneys, and the number of cases of scrotal cancer subsequently decreased (Waldron, 1983).

Increased protection

Exposure can also be minimized through the use of protective equipment, such as masks and protective clothing. For example, scrotal cancer was rare in sweeps in continental Europe and Scotland, where protective clothing was more widely used than in England and Wales (Doll, 1975; Waldron, 1983). A related approach is to impose protective hygiene measures. Three years after Pott's 1775 report, rules were introduced in Denmark requiring sweeps to take a daily bath, and since the start of this century Swedish sweeps have had the right to take a bath during working hours at the end of each day (Swerdlow, 1990). Nevertheless, steelworkers in the USA still experience an excess risk from exposure to coke-oven fumes—essentially the same exposures that Pott discovered were carcinogenic 200 years ago (Wagoner, 1976). Protective equipment has been introduced in numerous cases in developing countries, but use is often low because of the discomfort of wearing it in hot, humid climates.

Surveillance and education

An effective overall strategy in the control and prevention of exposure to occupational carcinogens generally involves a combination of approaches, including monitoring of exposures. One interesting example of such an approach is a Finnish registry which has as its objectives to increase awareness about carcinogens, to evaluate exposure at individual workplaces and to stimulate preventive measures (Alho *et al.*, 1988; Heikkila & Kauppinen, 1992). The register was established after ratification of ILO Convention No. 137 (see Chapter 9) and appears to be the only such national register currently in existence. It contains information on both workplaces and exposed workers (Kerva & Partanen, 1981), and all employers are required to maintain and update their files on employees exposed to carcinogens and to supply the information to the register. Regional labour inspectorates have legal power to order reports on exposure, and manufacturers and importers of any products containing carcinogens on the registry list must put warning labels on their products. Coverage of the exposed work-force appears to be only about one-third complete, however, and the number of workers reported in 1987 accounted for 0.6% of the total work-force (Heikkila & Kauppinen, 1992). Nevertheless, the system appears to have been at least partially successful in decreasing carcinogenic exposures in the workplace. For example, Alho *et al.* (1988) reported that hydrazine was previously widely used as an anticorrosive agent at power plants but that there had been a decline in its use which coincided with establishment of the registry system.

There are a number of analogous, but less comprehensive, programmes in developing countries.

Xue (1987) reported a dramatic decrease in the incidence of pesticide poisonings in Ho-Zhe District, China, as a result of education campaigns (Partanen & Kurppa, 1991). The cumulative incidence of occupational pesticide poisoning fell from 0.71% in 1981 to 0.021% in 1983.

A programme to survey workers exposed to organophosphate and carbamate pesticides was instituted in the Colombian province of Antioquia in 1981 by the Servicio Seccional de Salud (Forget, 1991). The proportion of workers with subnormal levels of acetylcholinesterase fell from 47% in 1981 to 24% in 1982 and 16% in 1984. This reduction was attributed to the concomitant education campaign.

In Egypt, a programme for studying occupational health problems was established with the help of the US National Institute for Occupational Safety and Health and the US Environmental Protection Agency. Investigations were carried out on and services were provided to agricultural workers exposed to pesticides and workers exposed to natural dust and fibres. The first group is the largest sector of the active work-force in the country, representing one-third of the total, while the second group is the largest sector of industrial workers in Egypt (nearly half a million workers, representing 8% of the active work-force). Workers exposed to mineral dust in mining and other industries were also included in the programme. The incidence of pesticide intoxication increased during the years of the programme, and the increase was attributed to a continuous growth in the use of agricultural pesticides. In contrast, significant reductions were reported in the prevalences of byssinosis and silicosis in industrial operations: Byssinosis was reduced from 38% in the early 1960s to 15% in the early 1980s, due mainly to increased awareness of excessive exposure by management and workers and to improved industrial operations (Noweir, 1986).

A good example of efforts to develop research in occupational epidemiology is a pesticide health and safety programme developed in Nicaragua by the American Friends Service Committee. The programme exploited and supported an existing surveillance system within the regional Ministry of Health. A supplementary form for reporting poisoning with pesticides was developed and distributed through the health centres of the National Health Service. The reporting of pesticide poisonings rose immediately, and teaching modules for the treatment of acute poisoning were established. It was found that 161 of the 351 cases of poisoning reported were due to the insecticide Furadan (carbofuran) and that 110 cases were due to metamidophos. Furadan was marketed in a powder formulation that is prohibited in many parts of the developed world. The programme demonstrated the practicability and usefulness of a good surveillance system for identifying problems and for developing policy (McConnell, 1988).

The East African Pesticide Network Group has initiated a research programme to assess the health hazards posed by the handling, storage and use of pesticides on agricultural estates and small farms in Kenya, the United Republic of Tanzania and Uganda, with a view to developing strategies for the prevention and control of pesticide poisoning (Anon., 1992). This programme, projected to last 3.5 years, is financed by the International Development Research Centre (IDRC) of Canada and is executed by the Occupational Health and Hygiene Department, Uganda; the Kenya Medical Research Institute, Kenya; and the Tropical Pesticides Research Institute, United Republic of Tanzania, in collaboration with the Finnish Institute of Occupational Health. The research project will occur in four stages: (1) a one-year preparatory phase involving surveys of farms, estates and villages; (2) a one-year implementation phase focusing on exposure to organophosphate and carbamate pesticides; (3) a further one-year implementation phase focusing on exposures to organochlorine and pyrethroid pesticides; and (4) a six-month phase for the final analyses and publication of results.

Comprehensive approaches

The occurrence of occupational cancer depends not only on levels of exposure to carcinogens but also on biological absorption and individual susceptibility, which are in turn affected by more general environmental conditions, including income, nutrition, housing and sanitation. Thus, although the prevention of occupational cancer is often focused on limiting individual exposures to specific agents (as discussed above), the greatest progress can be made when such measures are part of a more general strategy to improve living and working conditions. Such a comprehensive strategy is not only the most efficient in terms of the narrow goals of preventing occupational cancer but will also have other health and social benefits. Such programmes must, however, be complementary to, and never a substitute for, strenuous efforts to reduce or eliminate workplace exposures.

The Chinese experience in relation to chronic diseases is particularly interesting. Primary health care has been administered at the workplace for many years (Quinn *et al.*, 1987). Before 1949, all equipment used in mining was primitive and simple, underground working conditions were dangerous and hazardous to health, miners' housing was deplorable and health services were inadequate. After 1949, efforts were undertaken to improve the health status of miners in China, and preventive measures were taken. A study of conditions at the Huannan coal mine showed that underground dust concentrations decreased from 266 mg/m^3 in 1953 to 1.3 mg/m^3 in the 1980s; during the same period, housing conditions, water quality, nutrition and sanitation all improved markedly, and the prevalence of infectious diseases declined (for example, the prevalence of hookworm infection declined from 62% in 1950 to 21% in 1981) (Yang *et al.*, 1985, 1986). A study on the cumulative incidence of silicosis in 26 603 workers exposed in seven Chinese mines and industrial plants over 18 years showed a decrease from 36.1% in workers employed before 1950 to 1.5% in workers employed after 1960. The average age at diagnosis and survival increased during the same period (Lou & Zhou, 1989).

Although many forms of occupational cancer are rapidly fatal once they have occurred, occupational health services can nevertheless play an important role in cancer prevention. These services are inadequate in most developing countries, and there is a severe shortage of trained personnel (see Chapter 1); however, most preventive measures do not require highly trained personnel, and simple measures of occupational illness can be used by lay people (Loewenson, 1993). For example, Hessel and Sluis-Cremer (1985) found that non-medical readers were able to screen chest X-ray films for silicosis adequately.

The strength of unions appears to be one of the main factors in the provision of adequate occupational health and safety measures (Elling, 1986); however, in many developing countries, unions are weak (Chapter 1) and play only a small role in occupational health and safety. For example, in eastern and southern Africa, only the Zimbabwe Trade Union Congress has established an occupational safety and health programme (Loewenson, 1991; Sekimpi, 1993).

International controls

Efforts at the international level have centred on controlling the transfer of hazardous industries and hazardous wastes. A parallel can be drawn with the sale of arms: there is a global agreement that manufacturing nations take responsibility. A similar approach could be taken for chemicals and industries that are banned in industrialized countries for environmental or human health reasons (see Chapter 2).

The Basel Convention was adopted by 116 countries and those of the European Union on 22 March 1989 (Tolba & El-Kholy, 1992) and entered into effect on 5 May 1992. The main points of the Convention are:

(1)   A signatory state cannot send hazardous waste to another signatory state that bans its import or to any other country that has not signed the treaty.

(2)   Every country has the sovereign right to refuse to accept a shipment of hazardous waste.

(3)   The exporting country must first provide detailed information on the intended export to the importing country.

(4)   Shipments of hazardous waste must be packaged, labelled and transported in accordance with international rules and standards.

(5)   The consent of the importing country must be obtained before shipment.

(6)   Should the importing country be unable to dispose of the imported waste in an environmentally sound manner, the exporting country has a duty either to take it back or find another way for the safe disposal of the shipment.

(7)   Illegal traffic in hazardous waste is criminal.

(8)   A secretariat is set up to supervise and facilitate implementation of the treaty.

Similar recommendations have been developed for regulating hazardous industries. Thus, Noweir (1986) argued that:

> The protection and improvement of workers' health and well-being, in particular, and of the environment and community at large should be the responsibility of the new enterprises accepted by a developing country. The cost of control equipment and supplies for personal protection of workers, as well as of the equipment necessary for the protection of the general environment, should be part of the original investment of capital and should be considered in any feasibility study of new industrial development ... the standards and practices of the country exporting the technology should be applied in the new facilities.

Castleman and Ziem (1991) developed the following recommendations with regard to the information that should be sought from potential foreign investors for the purposes of environmental review (unlike the Basel Convention, these recommendations are not legally binding, but have been proposed as guidelines for use by developing countries):

Information from foreign investors for environmental review

A. The foreign investor shall provide an Environmental Impact Analysis of the proposed project, including:

(1)   list of all raw materials, intermediates, products and wastes (with flow diagram);

(2)   list of all occupational health and safety standards and environmental standards (wastewater effluent releases, atmospheric emission rates for all air pollutants, detailed description and rate of generation of solid wastes or other wastes to be disposed of on land or by incineration);

(3)   plan for control of all occupational health and safety hazards in plant operation, storage and transport of potentially hazardous raw materials, products and wastes;

(4)   copy of corporation guidelines of the foreign investor for conducting environmental and occupational health and safety impact analyses for new projects;

(5)   manufacturer's safety data sheets on all substances involved.

B. The foreign investor shall provide complete information on locations, ages and performance of existing plants and plants closed within the past five years in which the foreign investor has partial or full ownership, where similar processes and products are used, including:

(1) list of all applicable occupational health and safety standards and environmental standards, including both legal requirements (standards, laws, regulations) and corporate voluntary standards and practices for the control of occupational and environmental hazards of all kinds;

(2) description of all cases of permanent and/or total disability sustained or allegedly sustained by workers, including workers' compensation claims;

(3) explanation of all fines, penalties, citations, violations, regulatory agreements, and civil damage claims involving environmental and occupational health and safety matters as well as hazards from or harm attributed to the marketing and transport of the products of such enterprises;

(4) description of the foreign investor's percentage of ownership and technology involvement in each plant location, and similar information for other equity partners and providers of technology;

(5) names and addresses of governmental authorities who regulate or oversee environmental and occupational health and safety for each plant location;

(6) explanation of cases where any plant's environmental impact has been the subject of controversy within the local community or with regulatory authorities, including description of the practices criticized and how criticism was resolved in each case;

(7) copies, with summary, of all corporate occupational health and safety and environmental audits and inspection reports for each location, including such audits and reports by consultants;

(8) copies of safety reports, reports of hazard assessment and risk analysis reports carried out with similar technology by the foreign investor and its consultants;

(9) copies of toxic release forms that have been submitted to governmental bodies (e.g. the US Environmental Protection Agency or similar agencies in other countries) within the past five years for all plant locations;

(10) any information considered relevant by the foreign investor.

Agreements on policy

C. The foreign investor shall submit a statement of corporate policy on health, safety and environmental performance of worldwide operations. This must include the corporate policy on laws, regulations, standards, guidelines and practices for new industrial projects and production facilities. The foreign investor shall explain how its global policy is implemented by: describing the staff responsible for carrying out this policy, its authority and responsibilities, and its position in the foreign investor corporate structure. Such descriptions will also include the name, address and telephone number of senior corporate management officials in charge of this staff function. The foreign investor shall state whether it follows the same standards worldwide for worker and environmental protection in all new projects; and, if not, explain why not.

D. The foreign investor shall agree to provide the developing country immediate access to the proposed industrial facility at any time during its operation to conduct inspections, monitor exposure of workers to hazards and sample for pollution releases.

E.   The foreign investor shall agree to train fully all employees exposed to potential occupational hazards, including potential health effects of all exposures and the most effective control measures.

F.   The foreign investor shall agree to provide the developing country with equipment to analyse workplace exposures and pollutant generation, including, but not limited to, all limits specified in A.(2) above, for the lifetime of the proposed project. The foreign investor shall agree that the proposed project will pay the cost to the developing country government for all medical and exposure monitoring during the lifetime of the proposed project.

G.   The foreign investor shall agree that the proposed project will fully compensate any person whose health, earning capacity or property is harmed as a result of the project's occupational hazards and environmental impacts, as determined by the government of the developing country.

H.   The foreign investor shall follow marketing safeguards as restrictive as those it applies anywhere in the world to ensure that workers and members of the public are not harmed as a result of the use of its products.

I.   If the foreign investor becomes aware of a substantial risk of injury to health or the environment from a substance it manufactures or sells in the developing country, a risk not known and disclosed at the time of this application, the foreign investor agrees to notify the environmental protection agency of the government of the developing country immediately of such risk. [This is similar to requirements under section 83 of the Toxic Substances Control Act of the USA.]

J.   The foreign investor shall provide the names, titles, addresses, telephone and fax numbers of its senior corporate officials charged with implementing environmental and occupational safety and health policies including plant design and operations, corporate inspections and review of plant performance and product stewardship.

UNEP has developed an International Register of Potentially Toxic Chemicals to identify all chemicals that have been banned or severely restricted by five or more countries and is currently preparing guidelines to assist countries in establishing appropriate legislation.

Concluding remarks

New occupational causes of cancer continue to be recognized in developed countries (for example, cadmium and beryllium were recently placed in IARC Group 1 on the basis of new studies), but this is an increasingly rare event. Despite the considerable obstacles to the prevention of occupational cancer, the situation in most industrialized countries is generally continuing to improve (although occupational hygiene standards are often relaxed in times of recession). The improvement in occupational hygiene standards in developed countries has been achieved partly, however, by the transfer of hazardous industries to developing countries.

As documented in this book, total occupational exposures to causes of cancer are increasing in developing countries as a result of transfers of hazardous industries and the establishment of new local industries as part of a rapid global process of industrialization. These increasing exposures, together with demographic changes, mean that the problem of occupational cancer will be of increasing importance in developing countries in the next few decades. The examples of international measures, national measures and local initiatives described in previous sections serve to demonstrate some of what can be achieved in the prevention of occupational cancer in developing countries; however, such measures must compete with constraints imposed by the debt crisis and 'structural adjustment' programmes, which mean that occupational health problems are regarded as secondary to the daily struggle for survival (Michaels *et al.*, 1985). Although there is much that can be achieved in the current circumstances, substantial progress in the prevention of occupational cancer in developing countries is most likely to come from political and economic changes, including changes in the relationship between developing and industrialized countries and changes in political and economic priorities.

References

Aksoy, M. (1985) Malignancies due to occupational exposure to benzene. *Am. J. Ind. Med.*, **7**, 395–402

Alho, J., Kauppinen, T. & Sundquist, E. (1988) Use of exposure registration in the prevention of occupational cancer in Finland. *Am. J. Ind. Med.*, **13**, 581–592

Anon. (1965) Bladder tumours in industry. *Lancet*, **ii**, 1173

Anon. (1992) East Africa Pesticide Network. *Afr. Newslett. Occup. Health Saf.*, **2**, 75

Castleman, B.I. & Ziem, G.E. (1991) Environmental review of industrial projects evaluated by developing countries. *New Solutions*, **Summer**, 75–76

Doll, R. (1975) Pott and the prospects for prevention. *Br. J. Cancer*, **32**, 262–272

Doll, R. & Peto, R. (1981) *The Causes of Cancer. Quantitative Estimates of Avoidable Risks of Cancer in the United States Today*, Oxford, Oxford University Press

Elling, R.H. (1986) *The Struggle for Workers' Health. A Study of Six Industrialised Countries*, Amityville, NY, Baywood

Elling, R.H. (1988) Workers' health and safety (WHS) in cross-national perspective. *Am. J. Public Health*, **78**, 769–771

Forget, G. (1991) Pesticides and the Third World. *J. Toxicol. Environ. Health*, **32**, 11–31

Heikkila, P. & Kauppinen, T. (1992) Occupational exposure to carcinogens in Finland. *Am. J. Ind. Med.*, **21**, 467–480

Hessel, P.A. & Sluis-Cremer, G.K. (1985) The use of lay readers of chest roentgenograms in industrial screening programs. *J. Occup. Med.*, **27**, 43–50

Kerva, A. & Partanen, T. (1981) Computerizing occupational carcinogenic data in Finland. *Am. Ind. Hyg. Assoc. J.*, **42**, 529–533

Loewenson, R. (1991) Workers' activities in Zimbabwe. *Afr. Newslett. Occup. Health Saf.*, **1**, 88–89

Loewenson, R. (1993) Socioeconomic trends and health in developing countries. In: *Proceedings of the NIVA Course on Occupational Health Research in Developing Countries, Stockholm, 24–28 May 1993*

Logie, D.E. & Woodroffe, J. (1993) Structural adjustment: the wrong prescription for Africa? *Br. Med. J.*, **307**, 41–44

Lou, J. & Zhou, C. (1989) The prevention of silicosis and prediction of its future prevalence in China. *Am. J. Public Health*, **79**, 1613–1616

McConnell, R. (1988) Epidemiology and occupational health in developing countries: pesticides in Nicaragua. In: Hogstedt, C. & Reuterwall, C., eds, *Progress in Occupational Epidemiology*, Amsterdam, Elsevier Science Publishers, pp. 361–365

Michaels, D., Barrera, C. & Gacharná, M.G. (1985) Economic development and occupational health in Latin America: new directions for public health in less developed countries. *Am. J. Public Health*, **75**, 536–542

Noweir, M.H. (1986) Occupational health in developing countries with special reference to Egypt. *Am. J. Ind. Med.*, **9**, 125–141

Partanen, T. & Kurppa, K. (1991) Epidemiologic strategies and methods in occupational health and safety with special emphasis on developing countries. *East Afr. Newslett.*, **Suppl. 3**

Pearce, N.E., Davis, P.B., Smith, A.H. & Foster, F.H. (1985) Social class, ethnic group and male mortality in New Zealand 1974–78. *J. Epidemiol. Community Health*, **39**, 9–14

Pott, P. (1775) *Chirurgical Observations*, London, Hawes, Clarke and Collins

Quinn, M., Punnett, L., Christiani, D.C., Levenstein, C. & Wegman, D.H. (1987) Modernization and trends in occupational health and safety in the People's Republic of China 1981–1986. *Am. J. Ind. Med.*, **12**, 499–506

Sekimpi, D.K. (1993) The transfer of knowledge and technologies in the field of occupational health to African countries. In: *Proceedings of the 24th Congress of the International Commission on Occupational Health, Nice, 26–30 September 1993*, pp. 159–165

Simonato, L. (1986) Aspects of occupational cancer in developing countries. In: Khogali, M., Omar, Y.T., Gjorgov, A. & Ismail, A.S., eds, *Proceedings of the 2nd UICC Conference on Cancer Prevention, Kuwait, 1984*, Oxford, Pergamon Press, pp. 101–106

Swerdlow, A.J. (1990) Effectiveness of primary prevention of occupational exposures on cancer risk. In: Hakama, M., Veral, V., Cullen, J.W. & Parkin, D.M., eds, *Evaluating Effectiveness of Primary Prevention of Cancer* (IARC Scientific Publications No. 103), Lyon, IARC, pp. 23–56

Tolba, M.K. & El-Kholy, O.A., eds (1992) *The World Environment, 1972–1992: Two Decades of Challenge*, London, Chapman & Hall

Tominaga, S. (1986) Spread of smoking to the developing countries. In: Zaridze, D. & Peto, R., eds, *Tobacco: A Major International Health Hazard* (IARC Scientific Publications No. 74), Lyon, IARC, pp. 125–133

Ushewokunze, C.M. (1982) Socio-economic impact of asbestos use (cost–benefit analysis) with special reference to developing countries. In: *Proceedings of the World Symposium on Asbestos, May 1982, Montreal, Canada*, pp. 231–235

Wagoner, J.K. (1976) Occupational carcinogenesis: the two hundred years since Percival Pott. *Ann. N.Y. Acad. Sci.*, **271**, 1–3

Waldron, H.A. (1983) A brief history of scrotal cancer. *Br. J. Ind. Med.*, **40**, 390–401

Xue, S. (1987) Health effects of pesticides: a review of epidemiologic research from the perspective of developing nations. *Am. J. Ind. Med.*, **12**, 269–279

Yang, M.-D., Wang, J.-D., Wang, Y.-I., Guo, P.-S., Yao, Z.-Q., Lu, P.-L., Gy, X.-Y., Dong, Y.-L., Lu, M.-X., Zhu, P., Yan, S.-G., Liu, Q.-P., Jiang, M.-C., Chen, Z.-Q., Fant, S.-Q., Ren, S.-Y., Shen, D., Qiao, T.-Y., Huang, F.-S. & Jiang, Z.-D. (1985) Changes in health conditions in the Huainan coal mine in the past three decades. *Scand. J. Work Environ. Health*, **11** (Suppl. 4), 64–67

Yang, M.-D., Wang, J.-D., Wang, Y.-L. & Chen, Z.-Q. (1986) Changes in health conditions in the Huainan coal mine in the past three decades. *Ann. Am. Conf. Gov. Ind. Hyg.*, **14**, 385–389

Yin, S.-N., Li, Q., Liu, Y., Tian, F., Du, C. & Jin, C. (1987) Occupational exposure to benzene in China. *Br. J. Ind. Med.*, **44**, 192–195

Appendix. Survey of information on legislation, exposures and industries in developing countries

E. Matos and H. Vainio

This publication is based on published information and also on a survey of the situation in developing countries, which was conducted specifically for this purpose. The countries selected for inclusion in the survey were all those in Central and South America, Africa and Asia, except Japan. The industrialized countries of Europe, North America, Oceania and the former USSR were excluded.

Questionnaires in one of three languages (English, French and Spanish) were sent in March 1992 to ministries of health and to occupational safety and health institutions in developing and newly industrialized countries all over the world, together with a letter explaining the objectives of the study. Mailing lists from ILO (CIS) and WHO were used. Furthermore, a letter was published in the *African Newsletter on Occupational Health and Safety* (Vol. 2, p. 23, 1992), and individual letters requesting relevant information were sent to 60 people. By June 1993, 29 countries had forwarded a total of 33 questionnaires (two questionnaires each were received from Cameroon, Cyprus, India and Thailand). Table 1 lists the responses by country.

The selection of chemicals to be investigated was based on IARC lists of human carcinogens (see Chapter 4). In preparing tables of occupations and industries that present carcinogenic hazards, however, exposures that have not yet been evaluated by working groups at IARC were also taken into account. The selection of chemicals was also determined by the extent of material from the countries examined. IARC and American Conference of Governmental Industrial Hygienists categories of carcinogens were added for comparison. In addition, exhaustive searches were conducted on the following databases: MEDLINE, NIOSH, CANCERLIT, CISDOC (ILO) and NIOSHTIC; and almost 400 papers were reviewed.

Table 1. Answers to questionnaires by June 1993

Country	Source of information	Information on			
		Legislation	Exposure	Industries	Disease
Latin America					
Argentina	IO/ILO	Yes	No	Yes	No
Brazil	MH	Yes	No	No	Yes
Chile	IPH	Yes	Yes	No	Yes
Costa Rica	ML	No	No	No	No
Cuba	IO	Yes	Yes	Yes	Yes
Guatemala	ISS	No	No	No	No
Peru	MH	Yes	Yes	Yes	Yes
Africa					
Angola	ML	No	Yes	Yes	No
Benin	MH	Yes	No	No	Yes
Botswana	MH	No	Yes	Yes	Yes
Cameroon	IF/ML	No	No	No	Yes
Ethiopia	ML	No	No	(ILO data)	No
Madagascar	ML	No	Yes	No	No
Nigeria	MH	Yes	Yes	yes	Yes
United Republic of Tanzania	ML	No	Yes	Yes	Yes
Zambia	OOHS	No	No	Yes	No
Zimbabwe	TU	Yes	Yes	Yes	Yes
North Africa and Middle East					
Bahrain	MH	Yes	Yes	Yes	No
Cyprus	ML/MH	Yes	Yes	Yes	Yes
Egypt	ML	Yes	No	No	No
Jordan	MH	No	Yes	No	No
Kuwait	MH	Yes	Yes	Yes	Yes
Morocco	MH	Yes	Yes	Yes	Yes
Turkey	MH	No	Yes	Yes	Yes
South-East Asia					
India	NIOH/ML	Yes	Yes	Yes	Yes
Mongolia	MH	No	Yes	No	Yes
Philippines	ML	Yes	Yes	Yes	Yes
Singapore	ML	Yes	Yes	Yes	Yes
Thailand	MH/ML	Yes	Yes	Yes	Yes

IO, institute of oncology; ILO, International Labour Office; MH, ministry of health; IPH, institute of public health; ML, ministry of labour; ISS, institute of social security; IF, insurance fund; OOHS, organization of occupational health and safety; TU, trade unions; NIOH, national institute of occupational health

Individual sources:

South and Central America

Argentina: Instituto de Oncologia, Universidad de Buenos Aires; ILO Office, Buenos Aires

Brazil: Ministrio de Salud, Instituto Nacional de Oncologia, Rio de Janeiro

Chile: Instituto de Salud Publico, Santiago

Costa Rica: Ministerio de Salud, San Jose

Cuba: Instituto Nacional de Oncologia y Radiobiologia, Havana

Guatemala: Instituto Guatemalteco de Seguridad Social, Guatemala City

Peru: Ministerio de Salud, Instituto Nacional de Salud Ocupacional, Lima

Africa

Angola: Ministère du Travail, Administration publique et Sécurité sociale, Département national de Sécurité et Hygiène du Travail, Luanda

Benin: Ministère de la Santé publique, Direction du Travail, Cotonou

Botswana: Ministry of Health, Occupational Health Unit, Gabarone

Cameroon: Ministère du Travail, Inspection médicale du Travail, Yaounde; Caisse nationale de Prévoyance sociale, Yaoundé

Ethiopia: Ministry of Labour and Social Affairs, Addis Ababa

Madagascar: Ministère des Affaires étrangères, Tananarive

Nigeria: Ministry of Health, Lagos

United Republic of Tanzania: Ministry of Labour and Youth Development, Dar es Salaam

Zambia: Zambian Organization of Occupational Health and Safety, Ndola

Zimbabwe: Zimbabwe Council of Trade Unions, Harare

Middle East and North Africa

Bahrain: Ministry of Health Directorate, Al Manâmah

Cyprus: Ministry of Health, Nicosia; Ministry of Labour, Nicosia

Egypt: Industrial Safety Institute (under the Ministry of Labour), Cairo

Jordan: Ministry of Health, Amman

Kuwait: Ministry of Health, Kuwait

Morocco: Ministère de la Santé publique, Direction de l' Epidémiologie et des Programmes Sanitaires, Rabat

Turkey: Ministry of Health, Ankara

Asia

India: National Institute of Occupational Health, Ahmedabad; Ministry of Labour, Directorate General Factory Advice Service and Labour Institutes, Bombay

Mongolia: Ministry of Health, Ulaanbaatar

Philippines: Department of Labour and Employment, Occupational Safety and Health Center, Quezou City

Singapore: Ministry of Labour, Singapore

Thailand: Ministry of Health, Bangkok; Ministry of Labour, National Institute for the Improvement of Working Conditions and Environment, Bangkok

Subject index

PUBLICATIONS OF THE INTERNATIONAL AGENCY FOR RESEARCH ON CANCER

Scientific Publications Series

(Available from Oxford University Press through local bookshops)

No. 1 Liver Cancer
1971; 176 pages (*out of print*)

No. 2 Oncogenesis and Herpesviruses
Edited by P.M. Biggs, G. de-Thé and L.N. Payne
1972; 515 pages (*out of print*)

No. 3 N-Nitroso Compounds: Analysis and Formation
Edited by P. Bogovski, R. Preussman and E.A. Walker
1972; 140 pages (*out of print*)

No. 4 Transplacental Carcinogenesis
Edited by L. Tomatis and U. Mohr
1973; 181 pages (*out of print*)

No. 5/6 Pathology of Tumours in Laboratory Animals, Volume 1, Tumours of the Rat
Edited by V.S. Turusov
1973/1976; 533 pages (*out of print*)

No. 7 Host Environment Interactions in the Etiology of Cancer in Man
Edited by R. Doll and I. Vodopija
1973; 464 pages (*out of print*)

No. 8 Biological Effects of Asbestos
Edited by P. Bogovski, J.C. Gilson, V. Timbrell and J.C. Wagner
1973; 346 pages (*out of print*)

No. 9 N-Nitroso Compounds in the Environment
Edited by P. Bogovski and E.A. Walker
1974; 243 pages (*out of print*)

No. 10 Chemical Carcinogenesis Essays
Edited by R. Montesano and L. Tomatis
1974; 230 pages (*out of print*)

No. 11 Oncogenesis and Herpesviruses II
Edited by G. de-Thé, M.A. Epstein and H. zur Hausen
1975; Part I: 511 pages
Part II: 403 pages (*out of print*)

No. 12 Screening Tests in Chemical Carcinogenesis
Edited by R. Montesano, H. Bartsch and L. Tomatis
1976; 666 pages (*out of print*)

No. 13 Environmental Pollution and Carcinogenic Risks
Edited by C. Rosenfeld and W. Davis
1975; 441 pages (*out of print*)

No. 14 Environmental N-Nitroso Compounds. Analysis and Formation
Edited by E.A. Walker, P. Bogovski and L. Griciute
1976; 512 pages (*out of print*)

No. 15 Cancer Incidence in Five Continents, Volume III
Edited by J.A.H. Waterhouse, C. Muir, P. Correa and J. Powell
1976; 584 pages (*out of print*)

No. 16 Air Pollution and Cancer in Man
Edited by U. Mohr, D. Schmähl and L. Tomatis
1977; 328 pages (*out of print*)

No. 17 Directory of On-going Research in Cancer Epidemiology 1977
Edited by C.S. Muir and G. Wagner
1977; 599 pages (*out of print*)

No. 18 Environmental Carcinogens. Selected Methods of Analysis. Volume 1: Analysis of Volatile Nitrosamines in Food
Editor-in-Chief: H. Egan
1978; 212 pages (*out of print*)

No. 19 Environmental Aspects of N-Nitroso Compounds
Edited by E.A. Walker, M. Castegnaro, L. Griciute and R.E. Lyle
1978; 561 pages (*out of print*)

No. 20 Nasopharyngeal Carcinoma: Etiology and Control
Edited by G. de-Thé and Y. Ito
1978; 606 pages (*out of print*)

No. 21 Cancer Registration and its Techniques
Edited by R. MacLennan, C. Muir, R. Steinitz and A. Winkler
1978; 235 pages (*out of print*)

No. 22 Environmental Carcinogens. Selected Methods of Analysis. Volume 2: Methods for the Measurement of Vinyl Chloride in Poly(vinyl chloride), Air, Water and Foodstuffs
Editor-in-Chief: H. Egan
1978; 142 pages (*out of print*)

No. 23 Pathology of Tumours in Laboratory Animals. Volume II: Tumours of the Mouse
Editor-in-Chief: V.S. Turusov
1979; 669 pages (*out of print*)

No. 24 Oncogenesis and Herpesviruses III
Edited by G. de-Thé, W. Henle and F. Rapp
1978; Part I: 580 pages, Part II: 512 pages (*out of print*)

No. 25 **Carcinogenic Risk. Strategies for Intervention**
Edited by W. Davis and
C. Rosenfeld
1979; 280 pages (*out of print*)

No. 26 **Directory of On-going Research in Cancer Epidemiology 1978**
Edited by C.S. Muir and G. Wagner
1978; 550 pages (*out of print*)

No. 27 **Molecular and Cellular Aspects of Carcinogen Screening Tests**
Edited by R. Montesano,
H. Bartsch and L. Tomatis
1980; 372 pages £30.00

No. 28 **Directory of On-going Research in Cancer Epidemiology 1979**
Edited by C.S. Muir and G. Wagner
1979; 672 pages (*out of print*)

No. 29 **Environmental Carcinogens. Selected Methods of Analysis. Volume 3: Analysis of Polycyclic Aromatic Hydrocarbons in Environmental Samples**
Editor-in-Chief: H. Egan
1979; 240 pages (*out of print*)

No. 30 **Biological Effects of Mineral Fibres**
Editor-in-Chief: J.C. Wagner
1980; **Volume 1:** 494 pages **Volume 2:** 513 pages (*out of print*)

No. 31 *N*-**Nitroso Compounds: Analysis, Formation and Occurrence**
Edited by E.A. Walker, L. Griciute,
M. Castegnaro and M. Börzsönyi
1980; 835 pages (*out of print*)

No. 32 **Statistical Methods in Cancer Research. Volume 1. The Analysis of Case-control Studies**
By N.E. Breslow and N.E. Day
1980; 338 pages £18.00

No. 33 **Handling Chemical Carcinogens in the Laboratory**
Edited by R. Montesano *et al.*
1979; 32 pages (*out of print*)

No. 34 **Pathology of Tumours in Laboratory Animals. Volume III. Tumours of the Hamster**
Editor-in-Chief: V.S. Turusov
1982; 461 pages (*out of print*)

No. 35 **Directory of On-going Research in Cancer Epidemiology 1980**
Edited by C.S. Muir and G. Wagner
1980; 660 pages (*out of print*)

No. 36 **Cancer Mortality by Occupation and Social Class 1851-1971**
Edited by W.P.D. Logan
1982; 253 pages (*out of print*)

No. 37 **Laboratory Decontamination and Destruction of Aflatoxins B_1, B_2, G_1, G_2 in Laboratory Wastes**
Edited by M. Castegnaro *et al.*
1980; 56 pages (*out of print*)

No. 38 **Directory of On-going Research in Cancer Epidemiology 1981**
Edited by C.S. Muir and G. Wagner
1981; 696 pages (*out of print*)

No. 39 **Host Factors in Human Carcinogenesis**
Edited by H. Bartsch and
B. Armstrong
1982; 583 pages (*out of print*)

No. 40 **Environmental Carcinogens. Selected Methods of Analysis. Volume 4: Some Aromatic Amines and Azo Dyes in the General and Industrial Environment**
Edited by L. Fishbein,
M. Castegnaro, I.K. O'Neill and
H. Bartsch
1981; 347 pages (*out of print*)

No. 41 *N*-**Nitroso Compounds: Occurrence and Biological Effects**
Edited by H. Bartsch, I.K. O'Neill, M. Castegnaro and M. Okada
1982; 755 pages £50.00

No. 42 **Cancer Incidence in Five Continents, Volume IV**
Edited by J. Waterhouse, C. Muir, K. Shanmugaratnam and J. Powell
1982; 811 pages (*out of print*)

No. 43 **Laboratory Decontamination and Destruction of Carcinogens in Laboratory Wastes: Some *N*-Nitrosamines**
Edited by M. Castegnaro *et al.*
1982; 73 pages £7.50

No. 44 **Environmental Carcinogens. Selected Methods of Analysis. Volume 5: Some Mycotoxins**
Edited by L. Stoloff, M. Castegnaro,
P. Scott, I.K. O'Neill and H. Bartsch
1983; 455 pages £32.50

No. 45 **Environmental Carcinogens. Selected Methods of Analysis. Volume 6: *N*-Nitroso Compounds**
Edited by R. Preussmann, I.K. O'Neill, G. Eisenbrand, B. Spiegelhalder and H. Bartsch
1983; 508 pages £32.50

No. 46 **Directory of On-going Research in Cancer Epidemiology 1982**
Edited by C.S. Muir and G. Wagner
1982; 722 pages (*out of print*)

No. 47 **Cancer Incidence in Singapore 1968−1977**
Edited by K. Shanmugaratnam,
H.P. Lee and N.E. Day
1983; 171 pages (*out of print*)

No. 48 **Cancer Incidence in the USSR (2nd Revised Edition)**
Edited by N.P. Napalkov,
G.F. Tserkovny, V.M. Merabishvili,
D.M. Parkin, M. Smans and
C.S. Muir
1983; 75 pages (*out of print*)

No. 49 **Laboratory Decontamination and Destruction of Carcinogens in Laboratory Wastes: Some Polycyclic Aromatic Hydrocarbons**
Edited by M. Castegnaro *et al.*
1983; 87 pages (*out of print*)

No. 50 **Directory of On-going Research in Cancer Epidemiology 1983**
Edited by C.S. Muir and G. Wagner
1983; 731 pages (*out of print*)

No. 51 **Modulators of Experimental Carcinogenesis**
Edited by V. Turusov and R. Montesano
1983; 307 pages (*out of print*)

No. 52 **Second Cancers in Relation to Radiation Treatment for Cervical Cancer: Results of a Cancer Registry Collaboration**
Edited by N.E. Day and J.C. Boice, Jr
1984; 207 pages (*out of print*)

No. 53 **Nickel in the Human Environment**
Editor-in-Chief: F.W. Sunderman, Jr
1984; 529 pages (*out of print*)

No. 54 **Laboratory Decontamination and Destruction of Carcinogens in Laboratory Wastes: Some Hydrazines**
Edited by M. Castegnaro et al.
1983; 87 pages (*out of print*)

No. 55 **Laboratory Decontamination and Destruction of Carcinogens in Laboratory Wastes: Some N-Nitrosamides**
Edited by M. Castegnaro et al.
1984; 66 pages (*out of print*)

No. 56 **Models, Mechanisms and Etiology of Tumour Promotion**
Edited by M. Börzsönyi, N.E. Day, K. Lapis and H. Yamasaki
1984; 532 pages (*out of print*)

No. 57 **N-Nitroso Compounds: Occurrence, Biological Effects and Relevance to Human Cancer**
Edited by I.K. O'Neill, R.C. von Borstel, C.T. Miller, J. Long and H. Bartsch
1984; 1013 pages (*out of print*)

No. 58 **Age-related Factors in Carcinogenesis**
Edited by A. Likhachev, V. Anisimov and R. Montesano
1985; 288 pages (*out of print*)

No. 59 **Monitoring Human Exposure to Carcinogenic and Mutagenic Agents**
Edited by A. Berlin, M. Draper, K. Hemminki and H. Vainio
1984; 457 pages (*out of print*)

No. 60 **Burkitt's Lymphoma: A Human Cancer Model**
Edited by G. Lenoir, G. O'Conor and C.L.M. Olweny
1985; 484 pages (*out of print*)

No. 61 **Laboratory Decontamination and Destruction of Carcinogens in Laboratory Wastes: Some Haloethers**
Edited by M. Castegnaro et al.
1985; 55 pages (*out of print*)

No. 62 **Directory of On-going Research in Cancer Epidemiology 1984**
Edited by C.S. Muir and G. Wagner
1984; 717 pages (*out of print*)

No. 63 **Virus-associated Cancers in Africa**
Edited by A.O. Williams, G.T. O'Conor, G.B. de-Thé and C.A. Johnson
1984; 773 pages (*out of print*)

No. 64 **Laboratory Decontamination and Destruction of Carcinogens in Laboratory Wastes: Some Aromatic Amines and 4-Nitrobiphenyl**
Edited by M. Castegnaro et al.
1985; 84 pages (*out of print*)

No. 65 **Interpretation of Negative Epidemiological Evidence for Carcinogenicity**
Edited by N.J. Wald and R. Doll
1985; 232 pages (*out of print*)

No. 66 **The Role of the Registry in Cancer Control**
Edited by D.M. Parkin, G. Wagner and C.S. Muir
1985; 152 pages £10.00

No. 67 **Transformation Assay of Established Cell Lines: Mechanisms and Application**
Edited by T. Kakunaga and H. Yamasaki
1985; 225 pages (*out of print*)

No. 68 **Environmental Carcinogens. Selected Methods of Analysis. Volume 7. Some Volatile Halogenated Hydrocarbons**
Edited by L. Fishbein and I.K. O'Neill
1985; 479 pages (*out of print*)

No. 69 **Directory of On-going Research in Cancer Epidemiology 1985**
Edited by C.S. Muir and G. Wagner
1985; 745 pages (*out of print*)

No. 70 **The Role of Cyclic Nucleic Acid Adducts in Carcinogenesis and Mutagenesis**
Edited by B. Singer and H. Bartsch
1986; 467 pages (*out of print*)

No. 71 **Environmental Carcinogens. Selected Methods of Analysis. Volume 8: Some Metals: As, Be, Cd, Cr, Ni, Pb, Se, Zn**
Edited by I.K. O'Neill, P. Schuller and L. Fishbein
1986; 485 pages (*out of print*)

No. 72 **Atlas of Cancer in Scotland, 1975–1980. Incidence and Epidemiological Perspective**
Edited by I. Kemp, P. Boyle, M. Smans and C.S. Muir
1985; 285 pages (*out of print*)

No. 73 **Laboratory Decontamination and Destruction of Carcinogens in Laboratory Wastes: Some Antineoplastic Agents**
Edited by M. Castegnaro et al.
1985; 163 pages £13.50

No. 74 **Tobacco: A Major International Health Hazard**
Edited by D. Zaridze and R. Peto
1986; 324 pages £24.00

No. 75 **Cancer Occurrence in Developing Countries**
Edited by D.M. Parkin
1986; 339 pages £24.00

No. 76 **Screening for Cancer of the Uterine Cervix**
Edited by M. Hakama, A.B. Miller and N.E. Day
1986; 315 pages £31.50

No. 77 **Hexachlorobenzene: Proceedings of an International Symposium**
Edited by C.R. Morris and J.R.P. Cabral
1986; 668 pages (*out of print*)

No. 78 **Carcinogenicity of Alkylating Cytostatic Drugs**
Edited by D. Schmähl and J.M. Kaldor
1986; 337 pages (*out of print*)

No. 79 **Statistical Methods in Cancer Research. Volume III: The Design and Analysis of Long-term Animal Experiments**
By J.J. Gart, D. Krewski, P.N. Lee, R.E. Tarone and J. Wahrendorf
1986; 213 pages £23.50

No. 80 **Directory of On-going Research in Cancer Epidemiology 1986**
Edited by C.S. Muir and G. Wagner
1986; 805 pages (*out of print*)

No. 81 **Environmental Carcinogens: Methods of Analysis and Exposure Measurement. Volume 9: Passive Smoking**
Edited by I.K. O'Neill, K.D. Brunnemann, B. Dodet and D. Hoffmann
1987; 383 pages £37.00

No. 82 **Statistical Methods in Cancer Research. Volume II: The Design and Analysis of Cohort Studies**
By N.E. Breslow and N.E. Day
1987; 404 pages £25.00

No. 83 **Long-term and Short-term Assays for Carcinogens: A Critical Appraisal**
Edited by R. Montesano, H. Bartsch, H. Vainio, J. Wilbourn and H. Yamasaki
1986; 575 pages £37.00

No. 84 **The Relevance of *N*-Nitroso Compounds to Human Cancer: Exposure and Mechanisms**
Edited by H. Bartsch, I.K. O'Neill and R. Schulte-Hermann
1987; 671 pages (*out of print*)

No. 85 **Environmental Carcinogens: Methods of Analysis and Exposure Measurement. Volume 10: Benzene and Alkylated Benzenes**
Edited by L. Fishbein and I.K. O'Neill
1988; 327 pages £42.00

No. 86 **Directory of On-going Research in Cancer Epidemiology 1987**
Edited by D.M. Parkin and J. Wahrendorf
1987; 676 pages (*out of print*)

No. 87 **International Incidence of Childhood Cancer**
Edited by D.M. Parkin, C.A. Stiller, C.A. Bieber, G.J. Draper, B. Terracini and J.L. Young
1988; 401 pages £35.00

No. 88 **Cancer Incidence in Five Continents Volume V**
Edited by C. Muir, J. Waterhouse, T. Mack, J. Powell and S. Whelan
1987; 1004 pages £58.00

No. 89 **Method for Detecting DNA Damaging Agents in Humans: Applications in Cancer Epidemiology and Prevention**
Edited by H. Bartsch, K. Hemminki and I.K. O'Neill
1988; 518 pages £50.00

No. 90 **Non-occupational Exposure to Mineral Fibres**
Edited by J. Bignon, J. Peto and R. Saracci
1989; 500 pages £52.50

No. 91 **Trends in Cancer Incidence in Singapore 1968–1982**
Edited by H.P. Lee , N.E. Day and K. Shanmugaratnam
1988; 160 pages (*out of print*)

No. 92 **Cell Differentiation, Genes and Cancer**
Edited by T. Kakunaga, T. Sugimura, L. Tomatis and H. Yamasaki
1988; 204 pages £29.00

No. 93 **Directory of On-going Research in Cancer Epidemiology 1988**
Edited by M. Coleman and J. Wahrendorf
1988; 662 pages (*out of print*)

No. 94 **Human Papillomavirus and Cervical Cancer**
Edited by N. Muñoz, F.X. Bosch and O.M. Jensen
1989; 154 pages £22.50

No. 95 **Cancer Registration: Principles and Methods**
Edited by O.M. Jensen, D.M. Parkin, R. MacLennan, C.S. Muir and R. Skeet
1991; 288 pages £28.00

No. 96 **Perinatal and Multigeneration Carcinogenesis**
Edited by N.P. Napalkov, J.M. Rice, L. Tomatis and H. Yamasaki
1989; 436 pages £52.50

No. 97 **Occupational Exposure to Silica and Cancer Risk**
Edited by L. Simonato, A.C. Fletcher, R. Saracci and T. Thomas
1990; 124 pages £24.00

No. 98 **Cancer Incidence in Jewish Migrants to Israel, 1961–1981**
Edited by R. Steinitz, D.M. Parkin, J.L. Young, C.A. Bieber and L. Katz
1989; 320 pages £37.00

No. 99 **Pathology of Tumours in Laboratory Animals, Second Edition, Volume 1, Tumours of the Rat**
Edited by V.S. Turusov and U. Mohr
740 pages £90.00

No. 100 **Cancer: Causes, Occurrence and Control**
Editor-in-Chief L. Tomatis
1990; 352 pages £25.50

No. 101 **Directory of On-going Research in Cancer Epidemiology 1989/90**
Edited by M. Coleman and J. Wahrendorf
1989; 818 pages £42.00

No. 102 **Patterns of Cancer in Five Continents**
Edited by S.L. Whelan, D.M. Parkin & E. Masuyer
1990; 162 pages £26.50

No. 103 **Evaluating Effectiveness of Primary Prevention of Cancer**
Edited by M. Hakama, V. Beral, J.W. Cullen and D.M. Parkin
1990; 250 pages £34.00

No. 104 **Complex Mixtures and Cancer Risk**
Edited by H. Vainio, M. Sorsa and A.J. McMichael
1990; 442 pages £40.00

No. 105 **Relevance to Human Cancer of *N*-Nitroso Compounds, Tobacco Smoke and Mycotoxins**
Edited by I.K. O'Neill, J. Chen and H. Bartsch
1991; 614 pages £74.00

No. 106 **Atlas of Cancer Incidence in the Former German Democratic Republic**
Edited by W.H. Mehnert, M. Smans, C.S. Muir, M. Möhner & D. Schön
1992; 384 pages £52.50

No. 107 **Atlas of Cancer Mortality in the European Economic Community** Edited by M. Smans, C.S. Muir and P. Boyle 1992; 280 pages £35.00

No. 108 **Environmental Carcinogens: Methods of Analysis and Exposure Measurement. Volume 11: Polychlorinated Dioxins and Dibenzofurans** Edited by C. Rappe, H.R. Buser, B. Dodet and I.K. O'Neill 1991; 426 pages £47.50

No. 109 **Environmental Carcinogens: Methods of Analysis and Exposure Measurement. Volume 12: Indoor Air Contaminants** Edited by B. Seifert, H. van de Wiel, B. Dodet and I.K. O'Neill 1993; 384 pages £45.00

No. 110 **Directory of On-going Research in Cancer Epidemiology 1991** Edited by M. Coleman and J. Wahrendorf 1991; 753 pages £40.00

No. 111 **Pathology of Tumours in Laboratory Animals, Second Edition, Volume 2, Tumours of the Mouse** Edited by V.S. Turusov and U. Mohr 1993; 776 pages; £90.00

No. 112 **Autopsy in Epidemiology and Medical Research** Edited by E. Riboli and M. Delendi 1991; 288 pages £26.50

No. 113 **Laboratory Decontamination and Destruction of Carcinogens in Laboratory Wastes: Some Mycotoxins** Edited by M. Castegnaro, J. Barek, J.–M. Frémy, M. Lafontaine, M. Miraglia, E.B. Sansone and G.M. Telling 1991; 64 pages £12.00

No. 114 **Laboratory Decontamination and Destruction of Carcinogens in Laboratory Wastes: Some Polycyclic Heterocyclic Hydrocarbons** Edited by M. Castegnaro, J. Barek J. Jacob, U. Kirso, M. Lafontaine, E.B. Sansone, G.M. Telling and T. Vu Duc 1991; 50 pages £8.00

No. 115 **Mycotoxins, Endemic Nephropathy and Urinary Tract Tumours** Edited by M. Castegnaro, R. Plestina, G. Dirheimer, I.N. Chernozemsky and H Bartsch 1991; 340 pages £47.50

No. 116 **Mechanisms of Carcinogenesis in Risk Identification** Edited by H. Vainio, P.N. Magee, D.B. McGregor & A.J. McMichael 1992; 616 pages £69.00

No. 117 **Directory of On-going Research in Cancer Epidemiology 1992** Edited by M. Coleman, J. Wahrendorf & E. Démaret 1992; 773 pages £44.50

No. 118 **Cadmium in the Human Environment: Toxicity and Carcinogenicity** Edited by G.F. Nordberg, R.F.M. Herber & L. Alessio 1992; 470 pages £60.00

No. 119 **The Epidemiology of Cervical Cancer and Human Papillomavirus** Edited by N. Muñoz, F.X. Bosch, K.V. Shah & A. Meheus 1992; 288 pages £29.50

No. 120 **Cancer Incidence in Five Continents, Volume VI** Edited by D.M. Parkin, C.S. Muir, S.L. Whelan, Y.T. Gao, J. Ferlay & J.Powell 1992; 1080 pages £120.00

No. 121 **Trends in Cancer Incidence and Mortality** M.P. Coleman, J. Estève, P. Damiecki, A. Arslan and H. Renard 1993; 806 pages, £120.00

No. 122 **International Classification of Rodent Tumours. Part 1. The Rat** Editor-in-Chief: U. Mohr 1992/93; 10 fascicles of 60–100 pages, £120.00

No. 123 **Cancer in Italian Migrant Populations** Edited by M. Geddes, D.M. Parkin, M. Khlat, D. Balzi and E. Buiatti 1993; 292 pages, £40.00

No. 124 **Postlabelling Methods for Detection of DNA Adducts** Edited by D.H. Phillips, M. Castegnaro and H. Bartsch 1993; 392 pages; £46.00

No. 125 **DNA Adducts: Identification and Biological Significance** Edited by K. Hemminki, A. Dipple, D. Shuker, F.F. Kadlubar, D. Segerbäck and H. Bartsch 1994; 480 pages; £52.00

No. 127 **Butadiene and Styrene: Assessment of Health Hazards.** Edited by M. Sorsa, K. Peltonen, H. Vainio and K. Hemminki 1993; 412 pages; £54.00

No. 128 **Statistical Methods in Cancer Research. Volume IV. Descriptive Epidemiology.** By J. Estève, E. Benhamou & L.Raymond 1994; 302 pages; £25.00

No. 129 **Occupational Cancer in Developing Countries.** Edited by N. Pearce, E. Matos, H. Vainio, P. Boffetta & M. Kogevinas 1994; 192 pages £20.00

No. 130 **Directory of On-going Research in Cancer Epidemiology 1994** Edited by R. Sankaranarayanan, J. Wahrendorf and E. Démaret 1994; 792 pages, £46.00

IARC MONOGRAPHS ON THE EVALUATION OF CARCINOGENIC RISKS TO HUMANS

(Available from booksellers through the network of WHO Sales Agents)

Volume 1 Some Inorganic Substances, Chlorinated Hydrocarbons, Aromatic Amines, N-Nitroso Compounds, and Natural Products
1972; 184 pages (*out of print*)

Volume 2 Some Inorganic and Organometallic Compounds
1973; 181 pages (*out of print*)

Volume 3 Certain Polycyclic Aromatic Hydrocarbons and Heterocyclic Compounds
1973; 271 pages (*out of print*)

Volume 4 Some Aromatic Amines, Hydrazine and Related Substances, N-Nitroso Compounds and Miscellaneous Alkylating Agents
1974; 286 pages Sw. fr. 18.—

Volume 5 Some Organochlorine Pesticides
1974; 241 pages (*out of print*)

Volume 6 Sex Hormones
1974; 243 pages (*out of print*)

Volume 7 Some Anti-Thyroid and Related Substances, Nitrofurans and Industrial Chemicals
1974; 326 pages (*out of print*)

Volume 8 Some Aromatic Azo Compounds
1975; 357 pages Sw. fr. 44.—

Volume 9 Some Aziridines, N-, S- and O-Mustards and Selenium
1975; 268 pages Sw.fr. 33.—

Volume 10 Some Naturally Occurring Substances
1976; 353 pages (*out of print*)

Volume 11 Cadmium, Nickel, Some Epoxides, Miscellaneous Industrial Chemicals and General Considerations on Volatile Anaesthetics
1976; 306 pages (*out of print*)

Volume 12 Some Carbamates, Thiocarbamates and Carbazides
1976; 282 pages Sw. fr. 41.-

Volume 13 Some Miscellaneous Pharmaceutical Substances
1977; 255 pages Sw. fr. 36.—

Volume 14 Asbestos
1977; 106 pages (*out of print*)

Volume 15 Some Fumigants, The Herbicides 2,4-D and 2,4,5-T, Chlorinated Dibenzodioxins and Miscellaneous Industrial Chemicals
1977; 354 pages (*out of print*)

Volume 16 Some Aromatic Amines and Related Nitro Compounds - Hair Dyes, Colouring Agents and Miscellaneous Industrial Chemicals
1978; 400 pages Sw. fr. 60.—

Volume 17 Some N-Nitroso Compounds
1978; 365 pages Sw. fr. 60.—

Volume 18 Polychlorinated Biphenyls and Polybrominated Biphenyls
1978; 140 pages Sw. fr. 24.—

Volume 19 Some Monomers, Plastics and Synthetic Elastomers, and Acrolein
1979; 513 pages (*out of print*)

Volume 20 Some Halogenated Hydrocarbons
1979; 609 pages (*out of print*)

Volume 21 Sex Hormones (II)
1979; 583 pages Sw. fr. 72.—

Volume 22 Some Non-Nutritive Sweetening Agents
1980; 208 pages Sw. fr. 30.—

Volume 23 Some Metals and Metallic Compounds
1980; 438 pages (*out of print*)

Volume 24 Some Pharmaceutical Drugs
1980; 337 pages Sw. fr. 48.—

Volume 25 Wood, Leather and Some Associated Industries
1981; 412 pages Sw. fr. 72.—

Volume 26 Some Antineoplastic and Immunosuppressive Agents
1981; 411 pages Sw. fr. 75.—

Volume 27 Some Aromatic Amines, Anthraquinones and Nitroso Compounds, and Inorganic Fluorides Used in Drinking Water and Dental Preparations
1982; 341 pages Sw. fr. 48.—

Volume 28 The Rubber Industry
1982; 486 pages Sw. fr. 84.—

Volume 29 Some Industrial Chemicals and Dyestuffs
1982; 416 pages Sw. fr. 72.—

Volume 30 Miscellaneous Pesticides
1983; 424 pages Sw. fr. 72.—

Volume 31 Some Food Additives, Feed Additives and Naturally Occurring Substances
1983; 314 pages Sw. fr. 66.—

Volume 32 Polynuclear Aromatic Compounds, Part 1: Chemical, Environmental and Experimental Data
1983; 477 pages Sw. fr. 88.—

Volume 33 Polynuclear Aromatic Compounds, Part 2: Carbon Blacks, Mineral Oils and Some Nitroarenes
1984; 245 pages (*out of print*)

Volume 34 Polynuclear Aromatic Compounds, Part 3: Industrial Exposures in Aluminium Production, Coal Gasification, Coke Production, and Iron and Steel Founding
1984; 219 pages Sw. fr. 53.—

Volume 35 Polynuclear Aromatic Compounds, Part 4: Bitumens, Coal-tars and Derived Products, Shale-oils and Soots
1985; 271 pages Sw. fr. 77.—

Volume 36 **Allyl Compounds, Aldehydes, Epoxides and Peroxides**
1985; 369 pages Sw. fr. 77.—

Volume 37 **Tobacco Habits Other than Smoking: Betel-quid and Areca-nut Chewing; and some Related Nitrosamines**
1985; 291 pages Sw. fr. 77.—

Volume 38 **Tobacco Smoking**
1986; 421 pages Sw. fr. 83.—

Volume 39 **Some Chemicals Used in Plastics and Elastomers**
1986; 403 pages Sw. fr. 83.—

Volume 40 **Some Naturally Occurring and Synthetic Food Components, Furocoumarins and Ultraviolet Radiation**
1986; 444 pages Sw. fr. 83.—

Volume 41 **Some Halogenated Hydrocarbons and Pesticide Exposures**
1986; 434 pages Sw. fr. 83.—

Volume 42 **Silica and Some Silicates**
1987; 289 pages Sw. fr. 72.

Volume 43 **Man-Made Mineral Fibres and Radon**
1988; 300 pages Sw. fr. 72.—

Volume 44 **Alcohol Drinking**
1988; 416 pages Sw. fr. 83.

Volume 45 **Occupational Exposures in Petroleum Refining; Crude Oil and Major Petroleum Fuels**
1989; 322 pages Sw. fr. 72.—

Volume 46 **Diesel and Gasoline Engine Exhausts and Some Nitroarenes**
1989; 458 pages Sw. fr. 83.—

Volume 47 **Some Organic Solvents, Resin Monomers and Related Compounds, Pigments and Occupational Exposures in Paint Manufacture and Painting**
1989; 535 pages Sw. fr. 94.—

Volume 48 **Some Flame Retardants and Textile Chemicals, and Exposures in the Textile Manufacturing Industry**
1990; 345 pages Sw. fr. 72.—

Volume 49 **Chromium, Nickel and Welding**
1990; 677 pages Sw. fr. 105.—

Volume 50 **Pharmaceutical Drugs**
1990; 415 pages Sw. fr. 93.—

Volume 51 **Coffee, Tea, Mate, Methylxanthines and Methylglyoxal**
1991; 513 pages Sw. fr. 88.—

Volume 52 **Chlorinated Drinking-water; Chlorination By-products; Some Other Halogenated Compounds; Cobalt and Cobalt Compounds**
1991; 544 pages Sw. fr. 88.—

Volume 53 **Occupational Exposures in Insecticide Application and some Pesticides**
1991; 612 pages Sw. fr. 105.—

Volume 54 **Occupational Exposures to Mists and Vapours from Strong Inorganic Acids; and Other Industrial Chemicals**
1992; 336 pages Sw. fr. 72.—

Volume 55 **Solar and Ultraviolet Radiation**
1992; 316 pages Sw. fr. 65.—

Volume 56 **Some Naturally Occurring Substances: Food Items and Constituents, Heterocyclic Aromatic Amines and Mycotoxins**
1993; 600 pages Sw. fr. 95.—

Volume 57 **Occupational Exposures of Hairdressers and Barbers and Personal Use of Hair Colourants; Some Hair Dyes, Cosmetic Colourants, Industrial Dyestuffs and Aromatic Amines**
1993; 428 pages Sw. fr. 75.—

Volume 58 **Beryllium, Cadmium, Mercury and Exposures in the Glass Manufacturing Industry**
1993; 426 pages Sw. fr. 75.—

Volume 59 **Hepatitis Viruses**
1994; 286 pages Sw. fr. 65.—

Volume 60 **Some Industrial Chemicals**
1994; 560 pages Sw. fr. 90.—

Supplement No. 1
Chemicals and Industrial Processes Associated with Cancer in Humans (IARC Monographs, Volumes 1 to 20)
1979; 71 pages (*out of print*)

Supplement No. 2
Long-term and Short-term Screening Assays for Carcinogens: A Critical Appraisal
1980; 426 pages Sw. fr. 40.-

Supplement No. 3
Cross Index of Synonyms and Trade Names in Volumes 1 to 26
1982; 199 pages (*out of print*)

Supplement No. 4
Chemicals, Industrial Processes and Industries Associated with Cancer in Humans (IARC Monographs, Volumes 1 to 29)
1982; 292 pages (*out of print*)

Supplement No. 5
Cross Index of Synonyms and Trade Names in Volumes 1 to 36
1985; 259 pages (*out of print*)

Supplement No. 6
Genetic and Related Effects: An Updating of Selected IARC Monographs from Volumes 1 to 42
1987; 729 pages Sw. fr. 80.-

Supplement No. 7
Overall Evaluations of Carcinogenicity: An Updating of IARC Monographs Volumes 1-42
1987; 440 pages Sw. fr. 65.-

Supplement No. 8
Cross Index of Synonyms and Trade Names in Volumes 1 to 46
1990; 346 pages Sw. fr. 60.-

IARC TECHNICAL REPORTS*

No. 1 **Cancer in Costa Rica**
Edited by R. Sierra,
R. Barrantes, G. Muñoz Leiva, D.M. Parkin, C.A. Bieber and
N. Muñoz Calero
1988; 124 pages Sw. fr. 30.-

No. 2 **SEARCH: A Computer Package to Assist the Statistical Analysis of Case-control Studies**
Edited by G.J. Macfarlane,
P. Boyle and P. Maisonneuve
1991; 80 pages (*out of print*)

No. 3 **Cancer Registration in the European Economic Community**
Edited by M.P. Coleman and
E. Démaret
1988; 188 pages Sw. fr. 30.-

No. 4 **Diet, Hormones and Cancer: Methodological Issues for Prospective Studies**
Edited by E. Riboli and
R. Saracci
1988; 156 pages Sw. fr. 30.-

No. 5 **Cancer in the Philippines**
Edited by A.V. Laudico,
D. Esteban and D.M. Parkin
1989; 186 pages Sw. fr. 30.-

No. 6 **La genèse du Centre International de Recherche sur le Cancer**
Par R. Sohier et A.G.B. Sutherland
1990; 104 pages Sw. fr. 30.-

No. 7 **Epidémiologie du cancer dans les pays de langue latine**
1990; 310 pages Sw. fr. 30.-

No. 8 **Comparative Study of Anti-smoking Legislation in Countries of the European Economic Community**
Edited by A. Sasco, P. Dalla Vorgia and P. Van der Elst
1992; 82 pages Sw. fr. 30.-

No. 9 **Epidemiologie du cancer dans les pays de langue latine**
1991 346 pages Sw. fr. 30.-

No. 11 **Nitroso Compounds: Biological Mechanisms, Exposures and Cancer Etiology**
Edited by I.K. O'Neill & H. Bartsch
1992; 149 pages Sw. fr. 30.-

No. 12 **Epidémiologie du cancer dans les pays de langue latine**
1992; 375 pages Sw. fr. 30.-

No. 13 **Health, Solar UV Radiation and Environmental Change**
By A. Kricker, B.K. Armstrong, M.E. Jones and R.C. Burton
1993; 216 pages Sw.fr. 30.–

No. 14 **Epidémiologie du cancer dans les pays de langue latine**
1993; 385 pages Sw. fr. 30.-

No. 15 **Cancer in the African Population of Bulawayo, Zimbabwe, 1963–1977: Incidence, Time Trends and Risk Factors**
By M.E.G. Skinner, D.M. Parkin, A.P. Vizcaino and A. Ndhlovu
1993; 123 pages Sw. fr. 30.-

No. 16 **Cancer in Thailand, 1988–1991**
By V. Vatanasapt, N. Martin, H. Sriplung, K. Vindavijak, S. Sontipong, S. Sriamporn, D.M. Parkin and J. Ferlay
1993; 164 pages Sw. fr. 30.-

No. 18 **Intervention Trials for Cancer Prevention**
By E. Buiatti
1994; 52 pages Sw. fr. 30.-

No. 19 **Comparability and Quality Control in Cancer Registration**
By D.M. Parkin, V.W. Chen, J. Ferlay, J. Galceran, H.H. Storm and S.L. Whelan
1994; 110 pages plus diskette
Sw. fr. 40.-

No. 20 **Epidémiologie du cancer dans les pays de langue latine**
1994; 346 pages Sw. fr. 30.-

No. 21 **ICD Conversion Programs for Cancer**
By J. Ferlay
1994; 24 pages plus diskette
Sw. fr. 30.-

DIRECTORY OF AGENTS BEING TESTED FOR CARCINOGENICITY (Until Vol. 13 Information Bulletin on the Survey of Chemicals Being Tested for Carcinogenicity)*

No. 8 Edited by M.-J. Ghess, H. Bartsch and L. Tomatis
1979; 604 pages Sw. fr. 40.-

No. 9 Edited by M.-J. Ghess, J.D. Wilbourn, H. Bartsch and L. Tomatis
1981; 294 pages Sw. fr. 41.-

No. 10 Edited by M.-J. Ghess, J.D. Wilbourn and H. Bartsch
1982; 362 pages Sw. fr. 42.-

No. 11 Edited by M.-J. Ghess, J.D. Wilbourn, H. Vainio and H. Bartsch
1984; 362 pages Sw. fr. 50.-

No. 12 Edited by M.-J. Ghess, J.D. Wilbourn, A. Tossavainen and H Vainio
1986; 385 pages Sw. fr. 50.-

No. 13 Edited by M.-J. Ghess, J.D. Wilbourn and A. Aitio 1988; 404 pages Sw. fr. 43.-

No. 14 Edited by M.-J. Ghess, J.D. Wilbourn and H. Vainio
1990; 370 pages Sw. fr. 45.-

No. 15 Edited by M.-J. Ghess, J.D. Wilbourn and H. Vainio
1992; 318 pages Sw. fr. 45.-

No. 16 Edited by M.-J. Ghess, J.D. Wilbourn and H. Vainio
1994; 294 pages Sw. fr. 50.-

NON-SERIAL PUBLICATIONS

Alcool et Cancer†
By A. Tuyns (in French only)
1978; 42 pages Fr. fr. 35.-

Cancer Morbidity and Causes of Death Among Danish Brewery Workers†
By O.M. Jensen
1980; 143 pages Fr. fr. 75.-

Directory of Computer Systems Used in Cancer Registries†
By H.R. Menck and D.M. Parkin
1986; 236 pages Fr. fr. 50.-

Facts and Figures of Cancer in the European Community*
Edited by J. Estève, A. Kricker, J. Ferlay and D.M. Parkin
1993; 52 pages Sw. fr. 10.-

* Available from booksellers through the network of WHO Sales agents.

† Available directly from IARC